Melanoma Mama
On Life, Death, and Tent Camping

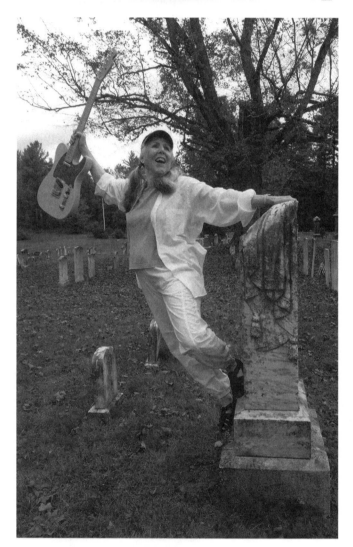

Constance Emerson Crooker

Dedication

In loving memory of my two primary caregivers
my beloved late mother
Elizabeth MacGregor Crooker Bates
1919 – 2011
and my caring, sweet stepfather
Dr. Frank Bates
who died of an undiagnosed chronic
lung disease in May of 2011

◇◇◇◇◇

Chapter One

I almost died of cancer. But I didn't. Not yet, anyway. Melanoma, the most vicious of the skin cancers, is one sneaky customer. The doctors warn that it is doing its best to outsmart my immune system. Mine is late-stage melanoma, so I am not considered cured. Nasty cancer cells lurk, awaiting their chance to proliferate madly. But lately, the score has been immune system one, cancer zero. The prognosis went from, "Get your affairs in order," to, "You have maybe twenty more years." I did the math. Sixty-three, plus twenty. That makes eighty-three. Woo-hoo. I'll take that.

The day I heard that my cancer treatments were holding the beast at bay I rejoiced with abandon. The Grim Reaper had been sneaking in my door. He had tiptoed over the threshold with his chortle and his musty stench. We had stared each other down. For several years I'd been drooping from cancer-caused anemia. For six months I'd been bombarded by cancer treatments concocted by the Marquis de Sade. For several weeks I lay nearly lifeless on my couch while I drifted in shadowy numbness. So, as I left the doctor's office that day, dancing in the hallway and whooping it up, I thrust my middle finger skyward and shouted, "Fuck the Grim Reaper."

I've been given what few Stage IV melanoma patients have received. Another crack at life. People want to know what that's like. How does it feel to go from shutting down, writing your will, and giving away precious possessions, to shopping for new clothes because now you'll have time to wear them?

I certainly wallow in joy more than ever. But where do I store my lingering doubt while living from scan to scan in dread of sudden bad news? Can I thrive while death lurks? Can I learn to embrace uncertainty?

I once wrote a story of which I'm now ashamed, because in it, I lied. I was in high school then, hospitalized for minor surgery, and assigned to an open ward with rows of beds. One night, the nurses quietly hovered over an old woman in the bed across from mine. Under cloak of darkness, they surreptitiously wheeled her out. One lone woman had died in the night. Just that day I had been talking to her. That mystery–how life courses through you, then suddenly ends–gnawed at me, so I wrote about it.

I wrote for a church youth magazine, and I manufactured a tearful husband, a Bible, and a sweet smile on the woman's peaceful face. It was all a lie, and I apologize now for telling it. She was alone. No husband. No Bible. No sweet smile.

We should never lie about death. The stories we fabricate to comfort ourselves and others aren't fair to the dying, to the deceased, or to ourselves. We'll all take that last step, and we'll look desperately for guidance. Will terror overwhelm us? Will agony crush us? Will we be robbed of the quality of life long before physical death? Is there a correct way to die? Should we peacefully accept death or should we rage against the dying of the light? Somebody, please, please, tell us the rules.

One unbreakable rule should be that we speak honestly. Having come all too close to death, I've glimpsed a few new things. I'll tell them here, and I promise not to lie.

When I received the fatal diagnosis in 2008, I considered whether to write about my ordeal, and I chose not to. Writing takes time, and time was in short supply. I wanted to enjoy the spaces between treatments with as much enthusiasm as I could muster. The hard parts–major surgery, devastating interleukin-2 treatments, debilitating radiation treatments–did not merit being relived in prose. Living them once was plenty. I needed to squeeze as much living as I could in the spaces between my dying.

Then, after more than six months of medical torture, came my reprieve. A midnight pardon granted, and my death sentence commuted. A last ditch round of radiation, intended only to alleviate my suffering, unexpectedly triggered a full bore attack on my inoperable tumor. Even with the good news, I'm still on probation. But I'm recovering. It has been gradual and often disheartening as I struggle to regain the fitness that once gave me such pleasure.

Before my decline, I could easily dance, ski, and hike. I could readily touch my toes. An exuberant zest for life came automatically packaged in a fit body. I had danced the Can-Can complete with cartwheels on my sixtieth birthday. (I danced a hip-grinding, Gypsy Rose Lee strip-tease too, but that's another story.) When I could no longer grab a full breath of air—when my joints all ached, and it became a chore to stand up straight–when I walked with a granny shuffle, the waves of discouragement were difficult to conquer. They sometimes still are, but I fight like a pit bull for my health.

I gradually discovered that I could begin to enjoy my former activities, even if in limited form, so I have been adding them back into my life. One thing I have loved is marathon, cross-country tent-camping trips; just me and my over-packed car, my AAA maps, and my wanderlust. So, six months after my last radiation treatment, when I had mustered enough energy to conceive of it, that's what I decided to do. I decided to see America up close and personal, getting sand between my toes and mud under my fingernails, because to know a place intimately, I believe you must get sweaty and roll in its dirt. You must let rain soak your socks and insects suck your blood. Smoke from campfires must sting your eyes. You must feel sticky hot and quivering cold. (But *don't* under *any circumstances* get sunburned.)

After radiation treatments, when I lay on my couch during what I call The Dreary Days, I thought I might never again see sunlit badlands or smell desert sage or hear the roar of waterfalls. Waking up to the songs of birds on the branches near my tent was a treasured memory, but I assumed I would never hear them sing again.

During my ordeal, I had purchased, for a mere ten dollars, my lifetime America the Beautiful National Parks Senior Pass. After age sixty-two, the pass allows free entry into national parks, monuments, and historic sites. That pass burned a hole in my pocket and in my psyche. From the moment I got it, I thought, "What if I die before summer, and my family finds it in my wallet, unused?" That little rectangle of plastic with a photo of a blooming cactus nagged and nudged me to get packing.

I improved through the summer of 2009, but not enough to take on the rigors of a long-distance camping trip. By early fall, I still had my doubts, but I thought I might have enough pep to enjoy it. Driving across the country by myself would be difficult, but with no time constraints, I knew I could manage. But camping in a tent? I've established a routine that seems, to me, like no big deal. But there's effort in all the bending and stooping to pitch a tent and bed down on an air mattress in a mini-dome in which you can't stand up. I also considered cold, rain, lightning, and all things that go bump in the night, not to mention the nighttime ups and downs that come with a 63-year-old bladder. But I recalled how I'd loved other long-distance camping trips, including the challenges, so why not try? In a pinch my credit card would buy the luxury of a real bed in a motel.

I yearned to see this land again, and to see it with the fresh eyes of recovery. It's a familiar cliché that a close brush with death can be a gift. They say it makes you live each day fully awake and aware. I can vouch for the fact that, after looking into the bleakness of the tunnel of no return, ice cream tastes sweeter, music sounds brighter, and the touch of a human hand thrills me with its pulsing warmth. I had already discovered the truth of this commonplace notion. So I longed to see the grand landscapes of this vast country with newly opened eyes.

I once attended a writing workshop with a marvelous teacher named Martha Gies. She taught us to approach our writing with the "traveler's mind." When you travel, you are more likely to notice details that you would miss in your daily life. You are looking for novelty and you open yourself to it, whereas in daily life, the familiar is what comforts us. She taught us to write always as if we were on vacation, seeking the new and the interesting. I have learned that I am happiest when I live the same way, as if on permanent vacation, always on the prowl for the fresh and surprising detail. Otherwise, life's a rut. And, as the saying goes, the only difference between a rut and a grave is the depth of the hole.

Thinking back on the worst weeks of my illness–the time after surgery, after interleukin-2 treatments, and just following radiation–the time when a nine-centimeter inoperable tumor in my chest fouled my lungs and blocked my esophagus so that I could swallow only mashed-up food–when I had yet to learn whether the harsh cancer treatments would benefit me–when I knew only that I did not want to push myself up off my couch to get a needed drink of water, I discovered one of the dreariest aspects of dying of cancer. It is really, really boring.

There *was* one thing I could do which gave me enjoyment, and that was to watch movies. So I stayed on my couch and watched three, four, and five movies a day. The concentration needed for reading was beyond me. Movies, on the other hand, would go on with or without my attention, and a snippet of dialogue would intrigue me even when I had napped through most of the movie–"Fasten your seat belts, it's going to be a bumpy night." (Thank you, Bette Davis.) I watched so many movies during that time on the couch that I felt guilty. I'd become a movie junkie. I thought, I get to lie around and watch back-to-back movies while other poor slobs have to go to work. Lucky me. But I suppose that stretches the concept of looking on the bright side.

So, in the winter of 2009, when I got the good news that my expiration date had been extended and that I had won the Melanoma Treatment Lottery, where the odds are about as unfavorable as the Publishers Clearing House Sweepstakes, I was determined to end the boredom of dying. I vowed to suck the juicy joy out of life.

I recognized the miraculous gift of a second chance. I hesitate to mention gifts and miracles, because it might seem like I'm dipping my toe in the baptismal font of religiosity. Trust me, that's not where this is heading. I'm not steeped in anyone's doctrine. But I do think about grace: when a person, through no personal merit, having done nothing more than any other terminal cancer patient, gets a second chance. There is a calm, a balm, a peaceful sigh of relief in feeling saved from certain doom. But call me skeptical–my best guess is that no misty, ghosty thingy sprinkles grace like Tinkerbell's fairy dust. I would never be rude enough to claim that God was protecting me above the many who have died of cancer. That's just wrong.

I'm not about to confirm any theology. I won't arbitrate the dispute over whether heaven consists of harps and haloes, phalanxes of virgins, or a tedious eternity with your dysfunctional family. I haven't a clue. I can only talk about life, and on that subject, I advocate living passionately and abundantly. Period. My purpose in writing this book is to show how much living can be done in the valley of the shadow of death.

So if you'd like to join me in a cross-country adventure, to see how a late-stage cancer patient seizes each day and packs it with geological marvels, wildlife adventures, and campsite calamities, then climb in and we'll take a freewheeling ride across this grand continent where we'll stand awestruck before the grandeur of life itself.

◇◇◇◇◇

Chapter Two

My basic purpose in driving across the country was to get from my home in urban Portland, Oregon, to our family farmhouse in rural New Hampshire where I am now writing this account. My more important purpose was to pour myself into America and to wrap America around me like a blanket. I needed to grow larger than myself and larger than my cancer.

I planned on taking almost three weeks because I wanted to avoid miserably long driving days and to sightsee at will along the way. Uncharacteristically, I drove partly on multi-lane, interstate highways. I normally choose only back roads through small towns so I can look around while driving. But I decided to travel in spurts, whizzing by some lovely countryside in order to pause at the great landscapes of the national parks. I'm sorry that some states got short shrift. I have learned that all states, including Oklahoma and Iowa have their scenic merits, although I have, on occasion, resorted to munching Cheetos to ease the boredom of vast stretches of not-much-to-see.

Everyone has a different style of traveling, so I won't pontificate on travel tips, but I started off with piles of predictable stuff: tent, sleeping bag, air mattress, cooler, dishes, camp stove, camera and binoculars, plus my trusty box of AAA maps, tour books and campground guides. And, needless to say, a big hat and lots of sunblock.

I will give only one travel tip right now. Listen up, ladies. Men, block your ears. Don't want to leave your cozy tent at night to go to the bathroom or the nearest bush? The best port-a-pee-pot in the world is a Folger's red plastic coffee can. No kidding. Do remove the coffee first. Inside your tent, you hold the handy handle and squat right over that puppy and then click the lid back on in case you kick it over in the night. This one piece of advice should be worth the cost of this book.

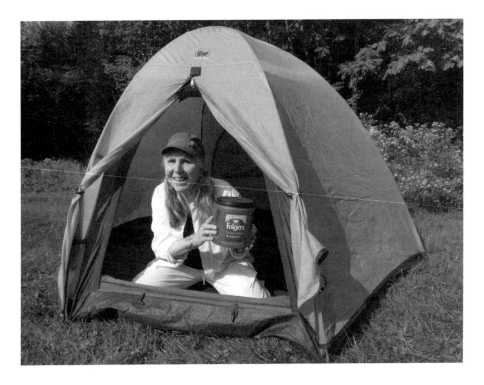

For men, it's been suggested to try a Gatorade bottle, but I have not had the privilege to observe how well that works.

Back to my pile of camping gear. On day one, I recruited my cheerful neighbor, Chris, to help me load my mounds of boxes and duffel bags into my aging Honda Passport. Chris is a worldly fellow, and is not easily taken aback, but I noticed the most peculiar expression on his face as he surveyed my possessions. I suspect the foolhardiness of what I was about to embark on was just dawning on him. His stunned look might have carried a touch of envy, but more likely he thought I was bonkers.

The first day was a breezy love affair with Oregon. As soon as I left Portland I was in the famous Columbia Gorge. This is a world-class destination for travelers who flock to see precipitous cliffs with cascading waterfalls galore. The gorge was carved out about 12,000 years ago during an ice age in which Lake Missoula (a modern name for a prehistoric lake the size of Lakes Erie and Ontario combined) burst its 2,500-foot-high ice dam. The entire lake roared westward over Idaho, Washington, and Oregon and got funneled through the gorge. Roiling with car-sized boulders imbedded in ice, the raging water smashed against the hillsides, gouging out the steep cliffs of the gorge in one sudden calamity. Or actually, a series of them. The ice age was in full swing, so the ice dam would form again, and within a hundred years would burst again and repeat the destruction. The geologists are still counting up how often this happened, but the series of floods carved out the gorge and dumped thick layers of soil into Oregon's Willamette Valley, which now boasts a rich, agricultural plain.

In the gorge, I drove past the Bonneville Dam. It spreads across the vast Columbia River in a phenomenal feat of engineering accomplished way back in the 1930's. Every time I drive through it I sing, out loud, Woody Guthrie's song, "Roll on, Columbia, roll on. Roll on, Columbia, roll on. Your power is turning our darkness to dawn, so roll on, Columbia, roll on." This giant dam still provides much of the power for the entire West Coast.

Of course, dams are controversial. The lakes that form behind them displace everything. Human communities, fragile ecosystems, and Native American petroglyphs all disappear as the water rises. Dams are good examples of both human ingenuity and human hubris.

There is talk now of removing the dams. Even with salmon

ladders, dams impact fish migrations and threaten the salmon's survival. It seems that hatchery-bred salmon lose some of their genetic hardiness, and are not a true substitute for the native salmon.

The salmon fisheries are themselves controversial. Everybody vies for a piece of the salmon action, including sea lions. During the salmon runs, you can stand near the Bonneville Dam and watch sea lions cavort in the current below the dam. They have something to cavort about, since they can easily snag their fill of migrating salmon. The fishermen hate the sea lions. Sea lions are big and fat. It's no secret how they got that way. The Oregon Department of Fish and Wildlife is perpetually trying to relocate the sea lions, but sometimes resorts to killing them.

Then there are the conflicts between the Native Americans and the rest of the fishermen. The tribes exercise their treaty rights to take salmon at their usual and accustomed fishing grounds "for as long as the rivers shall flow" and thus piss off the white guys who are subject to quotas. So it's the commercial fishermen versus the sports fishermen versus the Native Americans versus the sea lions. And it's the salmon versus the dams. It would take somebody much smarter than I am to referee that melee.

The gorge is wooded and, on the day I traveled through it, shared the rainy weather of Portland. As I drove east, the sun came out and the gorge flattened, first into the lush fruit orchards of Hood River, and then into the dry, treeless country where golden wheat fields spread across gently rolling hills.

On the car radio, I lost Portland's jazz and classical stations, and picked up Central Oregon's country and Mexican music stations. Stations that play authentic Mexican *ranchera* music, including *narcocorridos*, thrive in Central Oregon, where many Mexicans find agricultural work. The music has the classic sound of accordions with a polka-like beat and lyrics in Spanish laced with yipping aye, aye, ayes.

The *narcocorridos* are a fascinating sub-genre of traditional Mexican ballads. They tell of the daring exploits of drug runners outwitting the authorities. Occasionally they express repentance, but more often they glorify the drug dealers. This stems from a long Mexican tradition of romanticizing bandits who flaunt authority, as in the famous nineteenth century novel, *El Zarco* by Ignacio Manuel Altamirano.

As I drove along, one of the Spanish songs that caught my attention was a ballad with a twist. The singer describes the alluring pulchritude of his lover, and we expect the usual theme: "I can't help it. Passion is stronger than morality." But the sultry lover turns out to be the man's own wife.

I love to drive along the blue-green Columbia River with its tugboats and barges, its windsurfers and kiteboarders. Windsurfers stand on boards to which sails are attached. It takes great strength to hang on and scoot over the water, and even more strength to pull the sail up out of the drink when the windsurfer ditches. Kiteboarders get tugged along at breakneck speed by parachute-like kites, and the boarder sometimes goes airborne. I was driving where the bluff blocked the river from view, and was surprised to see this fellow flying through the air beside me. I hope his mother doesn't know what he's up to.

Forests of windmills adorn the bluffs at the river's edge. The windmills have proliferated in recent years in response to our need for alternate forms of energy. They look slim and graceful. A monumental, tapering pole supports three aerodynamically sleek blades that turn with slow ease. The insertion of these manmade giants into the landscape does not offend my eye. There is charm to their gentle dance above the wheat fields.

In places, there are tracks left by the wagon wheels of the

pioneers who drove across the prairies to settle in Oregon. The desert is slow to regenerate, and those tracks are still visible.

Past Pendleton, Oregon, home of a famous rodeo called the Pendleton Round-Up, the road climbs into wooded hills. Emigrant Springs State Park on Blue Mountain provides lovely campsites conveniently close to the highway–a bit too close for sensitive ears. The light was dimming and it was time for me to stop. I had forgotten that by mid-September the days would be noticeably shorter than in summer. During this trip I soon turned expert at making camp in darkness. I also imagined a balmy Indian summer, but, of course, at high elevations, even on warm days, the temperature can plummet at night.

I decided a campfire would be cozy, and I purchased a huge bundle of dry, pitchy pine by placing several dollar bills in a metal box nailed to a tree, and wheeling the wood to my site in a conveniently provided cart. The pitch helps keep the fire burning and its scent evokes memories of childhood campfires, rich and pungent.

The first evening by my campfire was idyllic. I sank into the lap of nature with no resistance. The pines rustled, the stars blinked, the friendly, muted voices of other campers floated my way, and the fire was just enough to take the chill off the mountain night. I had no guitar with me, but I felt like singing, so I sang *a capella*, at first timidly–more humming than singing– and then, without reserve. "Summertime, and the livin' is easy. Fish are jumpin'...," first sticking to the melody and then jazzing it up. I progressed to, "No one to talk with. All by myself. No one to walk with, but I'm happy on the shelf. Ain't misbehavin', I'm savin' my love for you, for you, savin' it for yoo-oo." Yeah, I really got into it.

Regarding my worries about sleeping on an air mattress in a tent, I wrote in my log, "I did well–minimum of aches and pains in lower back." That, of course means I had aches and pains, but ignored them. Cancer-caused anemia had fatigued me for several years, and repeated cancer treatments had clobbered me over and over. A few aches and pains were child's play.

My ordeal began nineteen years earlier, in 1990, when I went to my doctor for a routine check-up. He looked at a mole on my back and said, "That's coming off." I had been suspicious of that mole and had pointed it out to two prior doctors. They were unconcerned. Their lack of perspicacity delayed my diagnosis. This third doctor carved it off and shipped it to a lab. Uh oh. Trouble. It was "level three" melanoma, meaning it had grown deeper than the surface of my skin. It was described by the pathologist as "an ominous looking tumor." It had "some capillary involvement," meaning it might have begun to ship nasty cancer cells throughout my body. The doc used the word "metastasize," meaning spread. Who knows why doctors eschew the perfectly clear word, "spread" for the meaty mouthful, "metastasize." But then, I was a lawyer until my retirement, so who am I to squawk about opaque language?

I was in the prime of my law career and the news of the nasty mole felt like a punch to the gut. I was only forty-four years old, and I mentally played out my untimely demise over and over.

A friend gave me a tape that taught meditation and positive imaging techniques, and I grabbed onto it to calm myself. "Imagine yourself in a beautiful, peaceful place," the tape advised. It had a certain musical background that, to this day, brings up a memory of me sitting on a sunny rock by a gurgling stream, desperately trying to forget that I might soon die of cancer.

Although only marginally successful at calming my agitation, the tape helped me to focus on the fact that I was living. Such a simple concept. I'm still sucking air. Must mean I'm alive. So far, so good. That concept has served me well, like when I convinced myself that I was lucky to be watching so many movies during my hideous radiation. Focusing on life's pleasures has saved me from total despair. During the most grim moments, I've learned to grab whatever feeds my spirit. I cling to simple things like a friendly voice on the hospital phone, even though I warn the friend I probably won't remember the call because they've doped me to the gills.

So, after my original diagnosis, I had a surgical procedure called a "wide excision." They removed a big patch of skin around the original tumor site and checked for more ugly cells. I got my first good news. No more cancer cells. Then we had a tough decision. Do we watch and wait or do we clobber my system with chemo or whatever they were using in those days? The well-considered opinion at that time was to watch and wait. For years it seemed to have been the right decision. My quality of life was just ducky, I had regular blood checks and lung x-rays and skin checks, and ... nothing. One year, two years, three, four, and five. Zero, zip, nada. Boy, am I lucky. I beat that bad boy. I even outlived my first oncologist who died tragically in an airplane accident. (Now I warn my oncologists to watch out. I plan to outlive them all.)

So, unbeknownst to me, I had already won the Melanoma Lottery once before this. The cancer cells had, of course, secretly spread beyond the original site, and when that happens, they predict you'll take the dirt nap within about five years of diagnosis. The fact that I was not noticeably affected by my cancer for sixteen years is miracle number one. All that time, my immune system must have been tap dancing on those nasty cells. I've become a big-time cheerleader for my own immune system. "Push 'em to the left. Push 'em to the right. Come on system, fight, fight, fight."

$\diamond\diamond\diamond\diamond\diamond$

Chapter Three

In eastern Oregon, in the town of Wallowa, tucked at the base of the towering Wallowa mountain range, are real, working ranches. A college pal of mine owns one, and her daughters, all three Smith College graduates, have each put in time running it. They combine the wisdom of their forebears with modern ideas of sustainability to create the next generation in the all-important process of producing the food we eat. I called ahead and asked if I could visit on my way through. Daughter *du jour,* Nora said, "I'll be slaughtering a goat this morning, but you're free to drop by."

Slaughtering a goat? Uh oh. Ding, ding, ding. Mortality rings its death knell. Here one minute. Gone the next. Life. Death. Can I deal with watching a warm-blooded mammal meet its maker? I avoid killing insects. (Mosquitos, hear this–you are one big exception). Who am I to callously make life and death choices for some creature who has beat impossible odds in the evolutionary sweepstakes and is happily enjoying its moment in the sun? But I do eat meat. So that means I nurture my own squeamishness while somebody else plays hatchet man. Maybe it was time I faced up to where my food comes from.

It was a warm, sunny day and the road to Wallowa wound through Hells Canyon Scenic Byway along a clear, sparkling river and up a ravine that opens out to the high ranchlands that snug up to the dramatic Wallowa mountains. On the AAA map, that road shows little dot, dot, dots along it, meaning that it is an exceptionally scenic route. This route certainly earned its dot, dot, dots.

As soon as I arrived at the ranch I was greeted by Nora who

is lovely, lanky, and lean, with the shoulders of a linebacker from farm work, firefighting, and leading pack trains of elk hunters into the mountains. Her helper that day was a retired airline pilot from Alaska who globe trots in his private plane to hunt with his buddies, of whom Nora is apparently one. Bird hunting was on their afternoon agenda.

We immediately jumped into a field jeep to ride up through the pasture to mend a fence. While Nora and her friend stooped and propped fence poles and tugged and stapled barbed wire, the nearby llamas, cattle, and horses came clustering from curiosity, while a good old farm dog napped in the shade of the jeep. I stood photographing and pulling clean air into my radiation-damaged lungs. Waves of contentment swept over me. I was keenly aware of the privilege of living to see that lovely day.

We bounced through the fields back to the barn for the goat slaughter. Nora had agreed to provide a goat for a barbeque to be held by a group of forest-fire fighters. I took photographs—before and after pictures—throughout the process. But I was careful not to bond too much with Billy before the deed was done. He was a pretty, all-brown fellow, chosen because of the even color of his coat, which Nora planned to tan. He ran freely with the other goats in their comical joltings and bumpings as they wandered, unfenced about the ranch.

The process turned out to be intriguing, and I did, indeed, learn about where food comes from. The slaughter was swift, neat, and ethical. Here's how to properly slaughter a goat:

Separate Billy from the others and give him a bowl of grain. While his head is down, and he is happily munching his last meal, administer a quick bullet to the brain with a .22 rifle. (There was discussion over whether a pistol might have been better, but it was over in the other house.) Lights out occurs simultaneously with the gunshot cracking, and the goat feels nothing. There is subsequent muscle twitching in the legs, but the goat is already dead by then. The twitching is a result of muscles going limp and releasing tension.

Hang the goat upside-down by its hind legs and let it bleed out. (Yes, there is blood. It is red. It drips on the green grass where the dog licks it up.) Then slit the hide up the belly, and, starting from the hind hooves, peel it off in one piece with the help of a sharpened knife. Spread the hide slimy side up in the sun and thoroughly salt it for later freezing, then tanning. Slit the goat's belly, and let all the innards slide out into a waiting bucket, leaving a clean cavity that doesn't need washing. Save the heart in a bowl of cold water and promptly refrigerate. Wipe off visible blood with a damp cloth, but don't wash thoroughly, because a skein will form to protect the meat.

Not all of these procedures went without mild controversy between Nora and the older, slightly imperious airline pilot, who exercised a self-imposed duty to instruct the young lady who had already, herself, dressed out countless elk, deer, and farm animals. Nora was appropriately civil, and only occasionally mentioned her prior experience as they decided such things as whether you should gut the goat while it is still lying down, as you would an elk in the woods, or whether you should hang it up first, then gut it. And should you use a nearby barn bucket instead of a thoroughly cleaned house bowl to hold the heart? Should you wash off the blood with water, or should you just let the skein form? The discussions were businesslike and never descended to squabbling. They do teach those Smith College girls tact.

A death occurred that day. The goat was playing and romping, and then, in an instant, it was meat for the table. As businesslike as the process was, people did notice death. Several workers drove by the barn and saw the pearly flesh of the skinned goat and teased, "What terrible things you're doing to that goat." Then they drove off, laughing. It was like, see death, oh-my-god, crack a joke, drive on.

And when Nora was up to her wrists in blood as she knelt on the grass spreading heaps of salt on the hide, she reached out and patted the severed head of the goat, with its closed eyes and stubby horns. She said, "Hi, cutey. You look like you're just sleeping."

I told Nora that I was impressed with how humanely it was done. I said, "When my time comes, I'm going to tell the doctor to give me a bowl of Ben and Jerry's, and when my head is down, to let me have it."

The truth is, I have considered assisted suicide. Oregon law allows for it, but not, of course, with a bullet to the brain. A doctor must declare that you are within six months of dying. Two doctors must say you are mentally competent and are not depressed. (The law doesn't explain how you avoid depression when you know you have less than six months to live.) Then the doctors can authorize a lethal overdose of something or other. This is one option for avoiding suffering when the end is inevitable.

An alternative option is called hospice. Once you choose hospice, all treatments are intended to be "palliative" which means their purpose is to ease your suffering. With your consent, or the consent of your pre-authorized caregiver, all curative treatments are stopped, but you can have pain killers and tranquilizers—whatever you need to feel better, and you can keep taking medications for any other chronic diseases you might have. You simply stop taking curative treatments for your life-threatening illness.

I had not officially reached the stage of hospice, but my radiation treatments were intended to be palliative only. The idea was to shrink my inoperable tumor just enough to let me continue eating on my own, before the tumor would grow back again and completely block my esophagus. Instead, much to everyone's surprise, the tumor started shrinking and kept on shrinking and is still shrinking.

If my good luck doesn't hold, and I must choose between assisted suicide and hospice, I don't know which way I'll lean. I suppose it depends on how miserable I am. My inclination is to watch the movie to see how it ends. Some people die peacefully in their sleep, and others are awake and aware that they are dying. I think I want to be alert because I'm curious about everything, including what it feels like to die. But I say that now, when I'm not in pain. Regardless of what I might choose, I'm glad that assisted suicide is an option in Oregon and I applaud the legislators who braved opposition from those who base their arguments on understandable moral principles, but who, if they ever face hard, end-of-life choices, might readily change their minds.

Doctors, friends, and even some of my relatives have admitted to me privately that, at the end, when someone was suffering a slow, painful death, they have helped administer an extra dose of morphine to ease suffering and hasten the inevitable. Death by morphine overdose is apparently a common but unspoken practice even where assisted suicide is not legal. It is a shame that people must hide mercy killings or risk prosecution for murder, when, in fact, keeping a terminal and suffering patient alive can be supremely selfish. Medical providers bilk insurance companies for useless treatments. Family members who can't let go hold loved ones hostage to unendurable lives. Helping the dying to drift away painlessly can be an act of courage and selflessness.

After the visit with Nora, I spent the afternoon on a quiet ride through remote, northeastern Oregon. Another of AAA's scenic, dot, dot, dot highways goes from Enterprise, Oregon north to Lewiston, Idaho. You know you're in for a treat when the sign says, "Next gas 77 miles." The road winds over 4,000-foot wooded rises that overlook a dramatic canyon, and then twists down through parched landscape into a valley where the sparkling Grande Ronde River flows, then up again and across open ranchland to Lewiston.

Dusk was coming on as I settled in at the campground at Hells Gate State Park, just south of Lewiston. The campground sits beside the Snake River, which comes up out of Hells Canyon. The river flows to the north before taking a left turn into Washington, where it joins the Columbia River. Lewiston, in Idaho, is directly across the river from Clarkston, in Washington. Get the connection? LEWISton and CLARKston.

It was dark by the time I had pitched my tent and had blown up my air mattress and had arranged the bundles of things I need at night—a reusable shopping bag with toiletries and a towel which I carry to the campground's bathroom, a small satchel with nightgown and alarm clock and such, and my famous red Folger's coffee can.

I noticed that my lantern was attracting tiny bugs. They didn't seem to be biting, but they were clustering me to distraction, so I decided not to take out all my cook gear, but to throw together a sandwich instead, to avoid leaving the light on. I was wondering how I would entertain myself in total darkness, when my friendly neighbors invited me to come sit by their campfire.

It turned out to be one of those timeless evenings that only the hypnotic flames of a campfire can induce, where we chat, we laugh, we sit in silence, we toast marshmallows–with some turning golden brown, and others becoming flaming torches that end up with black, brittle crusts. We were three adults each recapturing our separate memories of marshmallow-filled childhoods in the out of doors.

This couple was cheery and chatty. They knew what an evening around a campfire is for. When the weather is warm and there's no rush to go anywhere and there's good company with faces lit by flames, the world beyond the surrounding circle of darkness fades away, and has reality only in the stories we tell each other.

These were what you might call average Americans——he, a manager of a motel chain, and she, a retired flight attendant. But there was nothing average about the size of their hearts. She was in a wheelchair, and he was patient and attentive to her, fixing her food, bringing her beverages, handing her marshmallows. She had suffered a stroke one year after retiring, and had recently had surgery on her curved-in leg. She hopes to walk again someday, but one arm will remain crippled. She laughed as she pointed to her bum arm, as if it were a naughty child that failed to mind her. Her tales of wilderness hikes in the past revealed an active, adventurous spirit, still alive in spite of her stroke.

She and I shared wheelchair stories. When you're in a wheelchair, some people are exceptionally helpful, while others don't seem to see you. I remember almost running over people in the airport. They would walk right in front of my wheelchair. I didn't know whether it was because they were higher up and hadn't noticed the low level of the chair, or because healthy people wear blinders to illness and injury. I do know that handicapped people notice and help each other.

Once, during The Dreary Days, I was shuffling with baby

steps up a hill at the Portland Zoo. A motorized cart for the disabled came by and stopped for me. I learned that it was not the driver who had spotted me struggling, but one of the handicapped passengers who had noticed my difficulty walking and had asked the driver to stop and offer me a ride.

The fireside subject shifted to Lewis and Clark who had passed this way on their famous expedition to the mouth of the Columbia River in the early 1800's. There are many sites all through the West that invite tourists to stand on spots that the explorers are said to have discovered. Of course, they didn't discover this land, since Native Americans have been here for thousands of years. As comedian John Wetteland says, "Columbus 'discovering' America is like a burglar 'discovering' your bedroom." The same can be said for the L&C gang "discovering" the West. And they may not have been the first *whites* in the area, either. Canadian trappers had been tromping about the West for some time, but since they weren't mapping it for the U.S. Government, they, like Rodney Dangerfield, got no respect.

Here at the Snake River, Lewis and Clark began their waterway journey to the mouth of the Columbia. But they almost didn't make it this far. They practically froze to death up in Lolo Pass, which is located in a rugged jumble of mountains between what are now Lewiston, Idaho and Missoula, Montana. From what I have gathered by reading Stephen Ambrose's excellent *Undaunted Courage* and by my peripatetic reading of roadside histories and visitors center displays, I have compiled my own unofficial history of the expedition, which I told around the campfire. Here's my version.

When Lewis and Clark and company reached the eastern side of these mountains, they told the local Indians that they needed a guide to help them to cross the mountains. They said they were looking for a big river that would lead them to a big ocean. So, along comes an Indian they came to call Toby. Old Toby is past his prime and is probably worried about how long his tribe will keep him in meat and moccasins, and here are these well-provisioned white guys who need help, so he pretends to know the way. "Sure, I know the way to the big river," says Toby.

So they start out over Lolo Pass, way too late in the fall, and they wind their way up and down over impossibly steep hills, and they lose a pack horse over the edge of a ravine, and the snow dumps, and they nearly freeze their feet off, and they're pretty much hopelessly lost and close to starving, but once you cross a divide and start following rivers downhill, you're bound to reach one that's larger than the others. That's how Toby, after twelve days of trouble, "guided" them to the Snake River.

With them on the expedition was the young Shoshone woman, Sacajawea, who was a great boon to the travelers, helping them find food and converse with various tribes, even though she had the extra burden of carrying her baby, Pomp, all the way to Oregon and back, *à la* Ginger Rogers who did every dance step Fred Astaire did, except backwards and in high heels. Sacajawea turned out to be a more useful interpreter than her ne'er-do-well Canadian husband, Toussaint Charbonneau, who had conned his way onto the expedition by claiming to speak languages he did not know. Sacajawea had been stolen from her tribe and had been traded around until Charbonneau won her in a card game. She was seen as extra baggage until her linguistic fluency was discovered and her status as sister of a chief was revealed. Once she joined the expedition, she remained loyal to it, and after it was over, Captain Clark helped raise Pomp, even sending him to college.

The only death was one soldier who died of a bellyache. Nobody got killed by Indians, who were hospitable all along the route, although I imagine some of the Indians' descendants wish they hadn't been so welcoming. The expedition members themselves killed two Indians who snuck into camp one night and pilfered something or other. I guess they figured they had to set an example, but the tribal backdraft forced them to flee for their lives.

The expedition itself was a huge, military boondoggle, over-equipped with big canvas tents, and a desk at which Lewis could sit and write his memoirs, and large, cast-iron cooking pots for feeding the nearly thirty men every day, and piles of junk no self-respecting camper would drag into the wilderness. In fact, Lewis and Clark had more comfortable accommodations than my own, because they could stand up in their tents.

And, although they are famous now, and have spawned a huge tourist industry, with people all along the Lewis and Clark trail claiming a piece of the tourist pie, they weren't even news in their own day. Lewis was supposed to write up his discoveries of new plants and animals from his journals, but he suffered bad moods, and had failed to keep consistent journals. Those he retained he never published, because he blew his brains out first. So all his discoveries were already well-known years later when his journals finally came to light. And the goal of finding a river route from the Missouri River to the Pacific Ocean was, of course, a failure, because of all those inconvenient Rocky Mountains in the way. So it wasn't until railroads came along that the goal of east-west trade on any scale was realized.

When Lewis came back east, he got into a kerfuffle with the army. At the time of the expedition, Lewis was a captain, but Clark was not. The army promised to promote Clark and pay him captain's pay retroactively when he returned from the trip. Then they reneged. So Lewis was on his way to Washington to have it out with them. He carried with him his satchel full of patent medicines which, in those days, probably contained opiates and cocaine and who-knows-what. So, at a wayside inn on the way to D.C., Lewis snuffed himself. Period. Nobody knows why, but I suspect that he was a manic-depressive self-medicating with toxic drug cocktails and wigging out with paranoia. But, as I say, this is an unofficial history told around a campfire. I told it my way, which includes saying "Indian" instead of Native American. It's shorter, it's traditional, and it highlights how geographically challenged Columbus was.

My new friend in the wheelchair got interested in Sacajawea and Pomp and said she would have to read up on them. Women are always drawn to that part of the story. The most noble character in the bunch was a kidnapped, sexually abused young girl who, in spite of that, helped the whole undeserving lot to survive.

◇◇◇◇◇

Chapter Four

In the morning, with none of those light-loving bugs to bug me, I lingered long enough to fix myself a bacon and egg breakfast in the cool morning sunlight under the pines. It was accompanied by an old family favorite, bacon-fat toast. The simplest way to keep breakfast prep to one pan is to make bacon first, then toast a slice of bread in the fat. Arteries, shut up. It's only an occasional campground treat.

Then I took a sunny, scenic (dot, dot, dot) drive, except that the Lochsa Wild and Scenic River Corridor turned into the Lochsa long and boring construction corridor. This is a twisting road that follows a lively river up into Lolo Pass. The road was being widened, and with good reason. I had passed this way once before and I remember seeing a gigantic semi facing nose-first in the river below. It had missed one of the many turns and had plunged straight down the steep bluff. I couldn't imagine how they would haul that huge honker out of there. So, this time, with road work all along this route, I repeatedly crept behind pilot cars in one lane, while construction crews took lunch breaks in the other lane. Federal stimulus money.

By the time I got to the visitors center at Lolo Pass, I was rummy. Bleary-eyed, I read more about the hapless Toby and also some bits and pieces about the geology of these mountains.

It seems that no matter how much I read about geology, it never sinks in. I can never remember during which multi-million-year time span an inland sea covered the area, or tropical vegetation made the place lush, or the mountains pushed up, or ice sheets smothered the whole shebang. I'm only left with a general impression that the earth has been around for a very long time, and that it keeps changing dramatically, and that human evolution is a hiccup in history. But I did pick up one bit of geological information that I have been chewing on ever since.

When there's an ice age, the ice can be thousands of feet thick (as thick as large mountains), and that ice weighs enough that it compresses the earth beneath it. The earth, after all, is only a thin crust of cooled rock that floats on a molten sea below. When the thick layer of ice melts at the end of an ice age, the pressure is released and the earth springs back up. That leaves room for gases to form down there. So, with the shifting earth and with underground gases wanting out, you get an increase in earthquake and volcanic activity following an ice age. I don't mean in the five or ten minutes following an ice age. I'm talking geological time. Our last ice age ended a mere ten thousand years ago. Hmm... Yeah. Hmm...

Coming down out of the hills into Missoula, I headed for a Mexican restaurant in the center of town. This is a historic area with cool eateries and shops and plenty of young people milling about. On the radio I heard this area referred to as the "hip strip." Sorry. I lived in the Haight-Ashbury area of San Francisco in 1967 during the famous "Summer of Love." That was the hip strip. Missoula, Montana in 2009? Nice try.

I drove on to make camp in the Beavertail Hill State Park, east of Missoula. The park is small, in a riverside setting with relaxing nature trails along the water. I could hear highway noise and trains going by, but I sleep with earplugs when needed.

I traveled the next day on I-90 through southern Montana. I must say, that for a multi-lane interstate, that road is plenty scenic with views of mountains all around. I stopped for gas in the dusty little town of Drummond, which features Mentzer's Used Cow Lot, a large corral decorated with an oversized, fake longhorn head with endless horns. I asked the mini-mart counter girl if she knew where there was a factory that made fake longhorn cattle heads and what the demand might be. She pondered, then admitted she didn't know. But she tried to be helpful.

Ever since hitting Missoula, I had been spotting a proliferation of so-called casinos, and was curious why there were so many, and why they were scattered about in truck stops and small taverns and such. I poked my nose in one to satisfy my curiosity. The manager told me that they are privately owned, but that Montana taxes them so heavily that they provide 90 percent of the state's revenue. If true, this is not that surprising. Jared Diamond, in his book, *Collapse,* describes Montana as essentially a failed state that would be in economic collapse were it not for the input of federal dollars. So Montana has apparently acquired a gambling addiction, which it hasn't been able to feed all that well with the downturn in the economy. According to this casino manager, the state is now jacking up property taxes to compensate for the loss of gambling revenue.

A larger problem with the Montana casinos is that the games are boring. There are only two types: video poker and video keno. Snore. The maximum payoffs are limited to something like eight hundred dollars. It wouldn't take long for a regular player to pump in that much money with little chance of hitting a jackpot. These games are sucker bait for the mathematically challenged. Oh, and they allow smoking. Get me and my bad lungs out of here, now. (As of October, 2009 the law changed. No more smoking. Not soon enough for my visit.)

I drove on, continuing to enjoy sunny September weather with temperatures into the 80's and crystal clear views of incredible western scenery with its rocky geology all hanging out and its vast blue skies and golden, reddish soils and crisp pines with sparse undergrowth. My car was climbing and climbing and soon the engine began to go all lazy from lack of oxygen. When I reached the top, a sign said, "Continental Divide." What a wonderful spot, where all the streams head either east or west. I wonder. If I were to pee at the pinnacle, would it flow to both oceans?

Another sign said, "icy spots," and I thought, maybe in February. Then suddenly, twist, jerk, slip. My car went out of control on what looked like smooth, dark pavement. It had been 80 degrees in the valley, for gosh sakes. But one shady spot of black ice woke me up fast. How absurd to survive cancer just to die in a car wreck. My poor family would be devastated, just when they've started to relax after all the nursing and toting me to doctors and hospitals. But the Grim Reaper was not lying in wait at the Continental Divide that day. The car soon corrected from its skid.

I pushed on to see if I could make it to Yellowstone National Park in time to make camp. I had been feeling well the first four days. The energy involved in pitching my tent and breaking it down, and in lifting boxes of camping gear from the car felt good. I was building needed strength. Plus I would stop often to rest. Driving alone, with nobody to spell me, I have learned to pay attention to sleepiness, hunger, and general fatigue. But this day, the rigors of the road crept up on me.

I still suffer side effects from my interleukin-2 treatments. IL-2 exhausts me. The exhaustion springs on me with no warning. The cycles of fatigue have faded over time, but I never know when I'll feel like a whipped pup. And both the interleukin and the abdominal surgery have left me with frequent gurgling in the gut. Bad bowels are debilitating. So I approached Yellowstone at suppertime feeling tired and, yes, grumpy.

Just past the tourist town of Gardiner, Montana is the impressive Roosevelt Arch, a stone structure dedicated by Theodore Roosevelt in 1905 to welcome visitors to the park. It stands alone, with the road on one side looking about the same as the road on the other, so its function as an entryway is difficult to perceive, but it's like a drumroll announcing, "You've made it." I received an extra welcome, for, posed in the road, right in the center of the arch, was my first elk. A real, live elk. Not a statue. Just past the arch a herd of elk grazed, pleasing the crowd of camera-toting tourists. But the onlookers outnumbered the elk by ten to one. Oh yeah. Yellowstone. A busy, popular place.

I approached the ranger's booth with my America the Beautiful pass in hand, relieved that I was near my goal. In a few miles I could settle into the campground at Mammoth Hot Springs.

Not so fast! Although it was a weekday in late September, and, as yet, no campground had been close to capacity, the ranger said that all park campgrounds were chock-a-block full. I must either make a reservation, or arrive in the morning to grab a site as another camper vacates it. The ranger handed me a list of places to stay in Gardiner. He said that if there were no vacancies there, I would have to backtrack almost sixty miles to Livingston. Ouch.

This is when I noticed that I was not entirely well. My ability to roll with the punches vanished. When my physical stamina goes, my mental agility also takes a hike. I felt confused and desperate. I began calling the Gardiner motels and campgrounds and checking them off the list. One after another, after another. I had gotten past ten when tears formed. I needed to lie down and rest. This was not optional. I kept asking whether the person at the other end of the phone knew of any other vacancy. Finally a fellow tipped me off to a place with one room remaining. I called and found it badly overpriced, but with a kitchen, so I could fix my own food. I snagged it.

This reveals the disadvantage of my freewheeling style of travel. I never plan, so how can I make a reservation? Something similar happened on a prior trip when I arrived late at night, after a long drive through an unpopulated region, and finally saw the welcoming lights of the first civilized burg in Idaho only to discover it was their annual Spud Festival, which apparently attracts thousands. That time I simply sat whimpering in the motel lobby, insisting that it wasn't safe for me to drive on, forcing them to cough up a room that they'd told me didn't exist. But that's the only other time I remember such a predicament. Taking my chances on camping and lodging almost always works out.

By the time I got to the motel in Gardiner, my stomach was so badly on the fritz that, even after three Imodium, I could only eat rice. All energy had left the building and I lay on the couch watching silly sitcoms. (Is that redundant?) I moped and sulked and felt sorry for myself. I pondered ash-canning the whole Yellowstone adventure, since my quick impression was that the park was overcrowded with boorish yahoos who take up all the campsites when they don't deserve them, because all they do is sit inside their giant R.V.'s watching silly sitcoms, instead of being out in nature like a true camper, such as myself, who, at the moment, was lying in a motel that smelled of Lysol, watching silly sitcoms, or did I already mention that?

As I lay on the couch, unable to motivate myself to take a shower or wash my one dinner dish, I pondered the wisdom of this adventure. I scolded myself for crapping out so easily, until I thought back over my ordeal and realized how far I had come. One year ago at this time I was recovering from extensive bowel surgery and could barely walk to the garden behind my mother's house. Only months ago, I was using wheelchairs and motorized grocery carts. I'll back up to describe what brought me to that state of disability.

During the winter of 2007, I first noticed troubling symptoms, starting with shortness of breath. I love to dance, and I was used to dancing vigorously and often. I danced the demanding lindy hop (a.k.a. jitterbug) and an improvised form of dance called ecstatic dance. In that winter, I noticed that the stamina that allowed me to dance long and hard was gone. Instead, I got dizzy and winded.

Then in the spring of 2007, I took off on a drive from Oregon to New Hampshire. Halfway across the country I felt like I was catching a cold. A rumbling, dry cough nagged me, and I tired easily. I expected to bounce back, and wondered why the cold lingered.

In New Hampshire, I belong to a hiking group called the Over the Hill Hikers. They divide themselves by ability into A, B, and C groups. I had always been an A hiker, tackling the rugged 4,000-foot peaks of New Hampshire. This time I found I could barely keep up with the C group. I waited for my cold to fade and my energy to regroup, but I got worse. One day, I didn't want to do laundry because it involved carrying baskets of clothing up and down one flight of stairs. I knew I was in trouble.

My mother took me to an emergency room and they discovered that I was badly anemic. When a number on a blood test gets below 12, they worry, and if it gets below 9, they give you blood. Mine was close to 6, or, as the doctor said, "half a tank low." They treated me with the first of a long series of blood transfusions.

They probed me top to bottom to find where I was leaking, but the mystery remained. I was bounced from doctor to doctor—more than five in one year. One doctor gave me a course of intravenous iron injections, which involved weekly trips to a chemotherapy ward, where iron dripped into my arm for three hours each visit. I used to chat with the chemo patients and count myself lucky that at least mine wasn't cancer. Little did I know.

I had a colonoscopy, an endoscopy, and I even once swallowed a camera that took pictures all through my digestive tract, transmitting them to the lab until I pooped the camera out the other end, where it continued to photograph the Portland sewer system. That test showed a raw, bleeding spot in my small intestine, but no treatment was recommended. Nobody expressed concern over my bout with melanoma eighteen years prior.

More than a year after becoming fatigued, I had reached the stage of needing transfusions every two weeks. Without them, I was bleeding to death. Then I had an allergic reaction to one of the transfusions. I panicked. If I could no longer receive my life blood I was done for.

I finally got referred to a gastrointestinal specialist, Dr. Steven Benson at the acclaimed teaching hospital, Dartmouth-Hitchcock in Lebanon, New Hampshire. At last I was in expert hands. Dr. Benson had just learned how to perform a new kind of endoscopy that could reach the difficult-to-probe spot in my small intestine. During my exam, he felt around my abdomen, then wrinkled his brow in concern. He ordered a CT scan to rule out any other cause of the bleeding. I wondered what he meant by "any other cause."

I showed up for the CT scan one morning. Barring problems,

the swanky new endoscopy would be performed that afternoon. I drank hideous goop and lay on a table that moved in and out of a doughnut-shaped machine. They said it would only take a few seconds to run the scan. They scanned my abdomen. Then there was a long pause. They scanned farther up. Then they paused again. They scanned farther up again, all the way to my neck. It took much longer than a few seconds. I knew something was amiss.

That afternoon, I reported for the endoscopy. Dr. Benson called for me and my parents to talk with us in the hallway of the operating area. There was a delay while somebody went to get chairs for us. The doctor apologized that there was no office there for a conference. It was clear the news was weighty, and it bothered him to deliver it in a bare, hospital hallway. He apologized yet again. He said that we would not be proceeding with the endoscopy. The CT scan showed two tumors. One, softball-sized in my abdomen, the other, also large, in my chest. He said it looked like lymphoma, "an easily treatable form of cancer." He referred me for a biopsy.

When we got the news, my usually upbeat 89-year-old mother startled me with her tears. I found myself hugging and comforting her instead of crying myself. Instead of sadness, I felt relief to know the cause after all this time. It wasn't until that night, alone, in my bed that I let loose a torrent. But I was not as terrified as I had been eighteen years before when I first faced my mortality with my original melanoma diagnosis. I thought that this time I had lymphoma, a treatable cancer, and I have seen many people survive cancer.

Then the biopsy came back with the news that it was melanoma–my old vicious cancer had returned and spread. My future, which I had always envisioned as stretching out through the years, became veiled by a grey curtain of uncertainty.

It takes resilience to absorb changing medical news without becoming overwhelmed. I did my best to keep pace with the sudden changes—mentally I shifted from being an anemia patient to a lymphoma patient to a melanoma patient in a matter of weeks. I eventually settled into a state of mind I call the Professional Cancer Patient where my job description was to put personal plans on hold and roll with the punches. Not that I didn't still hope and dream, but it became impractical to schedule anything more than doctors appointments. To get a sense of the emotional roller coaster ride I was on, here are excerpts from emails that I sent to friends and family that summer:

June 25, 2008: News from the northern wilds. I've seen lots of bears and lots of moose tracks, but no moose yet. I was supposed to fly home to Oregon today, but I'm up to my ears in doctors here, and didn't want to change docs, so until my medical mystery is solved (what causes my anemia), I'll be hanging out in New Hampshire.

July 9, 2008: There's light at the end of my tunnel of anemia. A specialist at Dartmouth-Hitchcock has a plan for me. It is a brand new kind of endoscopy (spiriul) that boldly goes where no endoscopy has gone before—— deep into the small intestine. Once there, if they find rotten spots (arterial venus malformations), they zap them so they stop bleeding (argon plasma coagulation.) No cutting involved. So I expect to have this done a week from Monday, two days before my 62nd birthday.

July 21, 2008: The procedure I was supposed to have today got canceled because a preliminary CT scan showed a tumor near the small intestine and another in my chest.

They appear cancerous, so I have a test on Thursday (July 24) to see what kind of cancer, so they'll know how to treat it. The likely suspect is lymphoma, which is treatable with a high rate of success. So I'm taking it one step at a time to see what needs to be done.

Mom and Frank are a great support to me right now, as are all of you. If you want to know what you can do for me, send me any oncology jokes you come across.

July 30, 2008: I know this email will seem an impersonal way to tell you my health news. I do want to speak personally with each of you if only to soak up all the love and support you've been sending my way.

I finally got the diagnosis that explains a year and a half of anemia. It is a recurrence of the melanoma I had eighteen years ago. So here's the plan they've outlined for me at the outstanding Dartmouth-Hitchcock Hospital (Lebanon, New Hampshire).

A week from now (Wednesday, August 6) I go for surgery to remove the abdominal tumor. Dr. Sutton will make a large incision, because he needs room to get the honker out. The in-hospital recovery will be about five days, followed by six weeks at home (Mom and Frank's house in New Hampshire) until the incision heals up.

Then, for the inoperable mass in my chest, Dr. Ernstoff takes over. He's a melanoma oncologist and has recommended that I be part of a study where they give you all the standard melanoma care (chemo and whatnot) plus a zippy new treatment. They send the tumor they removed to France where some hotshots turn it into a personal vaccine. Then, back here in New Hampshire they'll vaccinate me with my own cells. (Unfortunately they won't let me travel with my tumor for croissant and the Louvre.) Then they watch me for a year.

So it looks like my stay in New Hampshire will be an extended one, after which I'm still planning a trip to Italy, so I'm keeping up with my Italian studies.

When I was finally accurately diagnosed, all the missed opportunities for spotting my melanoma astonished me. I was furious at all the idiot doctors who had failed to order the simple CT scan that finally spotlighted the culprit. Plus I was angry that none of them noted a connection of which melanoma oncologists are well aware.

I have vitiligo, and have had it since 2002. Vitiligo is a condition where your skin fails to produce melanin, so you develop white splotches. Melanoma oncologists know that, in a patient with a history of melanoma this can be a sign that the immune system is battling a recurrence of melanoma. But they've apparently neglected to inform the rest of the medical community. Even my dermatologist, who checked my skin annually, and who knew of both my melanoma history and my vitiligo, had been unaware of this correlation.

About my anger. It lasted only briefly. Then I dropped it like a hot rock. I knew I was a sick little girl. The anger juices that churned in me felt poisonous. I thought that if I allowed that witches' brew of resentment to find a permanent home, it could interfere with healing. I'm a big fan of the serenity prayer, minus the invocation to the Big Guy. My version goes, "[God——deleted], grant me the serenity to accept the things I cannot change, the courage to change the things I can, and the wisdom to know the difference," or, in common parlance, if you can't fix it, don't sweat it. There was not one thing I could do to change my long history of missed medical opportunities.

I let my anger go with one big flush down the toilet of time.

People say, not possible. Anger is an emotion. You can't control your emotions—they come unbidden like internal tsunamis. True. I can't control my initial anger. But once anger surfaces, I can either cling to it, and nurse it, and get all juiced up on it, or I can let it fizzle out. I've noticed that nursing anger is seldom useful. It might help when fighting for a worthy cause. And rearing up on my hind legs can grab a person's attention when needed. But I knew that staying angry at my doctors wouldn't get me squat.

Seeing things from the doctors' side also helped. Doctors look for the most likely cause of a problem. I had bleeding in my small intestine. Most likely cause? Arterial venus malformations, which I picture as sores in the lining of the intestine. It's rare that anything outside the intestine would cause the bleeding, so nobody thought to look there.

I simmered down when I also considered what would have happened if they had discovered the source of the bleeding a year and a half earlier. The bleeding, even back then, was caused by a tumor that must have grown pretty large to do that kind of damage. Uh oh. Guess what. Stage IV melanoma. Same diagnosis. Probably the same treatments. I couldn't stew over missed opportunities when I had so much other medical news to stew about.

Dr. Ernstoff was the first to stun me with the seriousness of my situation. He told me the surgeon could remove the tumor from my abdomen, but the mass in my chest was "inoperable." We would have to treat that with either a standard regimen or a clinical trial, such as making a vaccine from my tumor. He let me know clearly that Stage IV melanoma is difficult to survive.

Nobody wants to hear the words "cancer" and "inoperable" in the same sentence. I asked Dr. Ernstoff, "Is there a Stage V, or is that the other side of the grass?"

He said, "There's no Stage V."

He encouraged me not to go by the percentages (my chance of long-term survival was miniscule) but to assume I would be one of the rare, lucky ones. In the meantime, I should get my affairs in order. A bit of a mixed message, I think.

So that's how I ended up in surgery in the summer of 2008. The surgeon removed the tumor, cut the intestine in two and sewed it back together again, minus the bleeding tumor. The surgery stopped the anemia, and that site remains cancer free.

The surgery packed a wallop. I was a dishrag for six weeks. My 89-year-old mother and my 83-year-old stepfather, Frank, nursed me constantly, not to mention their frequent two-hour drives to Dartmouth-Hitchcock. Thanks a gazillion, Mom and Frank.

Then I discovered I was not a candidate for the clinical trial where my tumor would have been shipped to France. A couple of other clinical trials also fell through. You must meet criteria for these trials, and I kept flunking their tests. I told Dr. Ernstoff that I wanted to stop fiddling with time-wasting tests and start treatment. That's when he clobbered me with interleukin-2. Then he clobbered me again with more interleukin-2. Then I got blasted with radiation. But more on those later. The point is, I was repeatedly subjected to the harshest forms of medical treatment known to modern science, and on top of that, I was sick from the cancer itself.

Toward the end, I couldn't drive myself to my radiation treatments. I qualified for handicapped parking. I used motorized carts in grocery stores and a wheelchair to navigate long, airport corridors.

So, by comparison, one evening of feeling tired after four long days of driving was nothing short of a miracle. As I lay exhausted on the couch in my Gardiner motel room, I told myself, "Quit yer bellyachin'." I let my fatigue and sense of disappointment ebb and flow while I rested, waiting to see what the next day would bring.

◇◇◇◇◇

Chapter Five

In the morning, the sun shone, the air was crisp, and I noticed with glee that I had a rodeo corral right outside my bedroom window. I'm in the Wild West now. My growly stomach had settled and Yellowstone seemed, again, like a splendid idea. I reached the campground by 8:30 a.m. and had my choice of sites for two nights. This gave me three full days to explore and goof off. With my parks pass, the park entry was free, and the campsite was half price ($7 a night), so I was finally reaping the benefits of my magic pass.

Part of my plan included reviving childhood memories. In 1959, my family, a mix of the ebullient Ozzie and Harriet and Leave it to Beaver families (with a touch of The Munsters— no family is *that* prissy perfect), packed up our sky-blue 1956 Plymouth station wagon for a camping trip from New England to Yellowstone. I was twelve. We saw the Badlands, Mt. Rushmore, the Bighorns, the Tetons, and Yellowstone. Now I planned to see them again, in part to recapture the joys and tribulations of family togetherness.

We had taken that trip because my mother, in the early 1930's, was taken by her parents on the same cross-country adventure, and she wanted her own family to see what she had enjoyed as a child. Her family took that 1930's trip because my grandfather, in the early 1900's had taken the train to Yellowstone and loved it so much that he wanted to show his family the marvels of the place. My hat's off to the National Park Service for keeping this treasure intact for generations to enjoy.

There are many ways to tour Yellowstone, which range from hurried visits to see crowded attractions like Old Faithful, to solitary, back country hiking on any of a thousand miles of trails *à la* Edward Abbey, whose classic outdoor saga, *Desert Solitaire*, inspires the intrepid to seek the wildest of the wilds. I am not a herd animal, so my style would normally lean toward Edward Abbey, but due to my limited energy, I fell somewhere in between, sometimes following the masses, and sometimes walking short distances into the puckerbrush.

Even if you never get off the beaten track, there's plenty to see. You don't have to search for wildlife. You must avoid crashing into it. On this trip, buffalo were the road hogs. Back in the fifties, bears stopped traffic to beg for food. A famous family photo features Dad holding an ax aloft while shooing a bear away from a food cooler. (Mom was like, wait, wait, I've got to get the picture.) Now the Park Service has finally convinced folks not to feed the bears, and I only saw three—a mother at the base of a tree and two cubs upstairs, rattling the branches. It is actually more thrilling to catch sight of truly wild animals that avoid humans than to trip over pesky moochers.

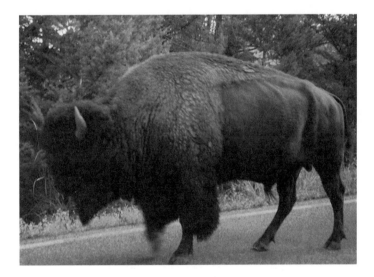

The buffalo don't mooch, because they prefer grass to peanut butter sandwiches, but they are everywhere in the park, in herds or alone, in their natural setting or wandering down the paved road. One curvy, mountain road was the only level spot carved out of a steep hillside, so a buffalo that ambled at a leisurely pace taking up one entire lane was unable to turn off on the steep slope to either side. Traffic was backed up for half a mile. I hope nobody was in a hurry. I wasn't. I snapped a photo as the buffalo strolled past my car. I rolled down the window for a better picture. Probably not smart of me. These animals are big. They have horns. I suspect they have a genetic grudge against our ancestors.

I should point out that I prefer the word buffalo to the one used throughout the park signage, which is bison. Bison is the more accurate scientific name, but so what? Common usage can trump scientific terminology, and "bison" lacks a romantic ring. Try singing, "Oh give me a home where the bison roam." It's missing a beat.

After my first day of touring, I wrote in my journal, "This morning, as I took off on my day trip, I rejoiced at being alive and present at this day's adventures." I also scribbled, "I saw a bunch of way cool stuff," proving that writers are not always eloquent in their first drafts. But it was true. I saw a bunch of way cool stuff.

I took a six-mile gravel road called Blacktail Plateau Drive, which is an alternate to the paved road. It forces you to slow down and notice. I stopped for views of distant mountains, and to examine roadside wildflowers, and to smell that western smell of pungent pines and sagebrush.

I checked with my binoculars to see if a dark brown rock was really a rock. It turned out to be the world's laziest buffalo dozing in the shade doing a perfect rock imitation except for its twitching tail. I thought of Ferdinand the Bull who preferred sitting under a cork tree to running and fighting.

Another shade sitter was a deer sporting an elegant rack of antlers. He nestled in the bushes right next to the Tower General Store at Tower Falls, which bustled with multilingual tourists all crowding to see the deer in the bushes. When nobody is shooting at these critters they could care less about our presence. This is their home and we're pesky transients.

I saw a coyote cross the road right in front of me. It was hefty, with a full, rich coat of grey-brown hair and a dark tip on its tail. It was either growing its winter coat, or it dines better than the scraggly Oregon coyotes I've seen. A handsome, self-confident fellow he was. I stopped to look at him, and he looked at me as if he owned the place, and who was I anyway? Oh yeah. He does own the place; and who am I, anyway?

I took a self-guided nature walk. I have to caution myself not to spend more time reading the interpretive signs than looking at nature, but I glean intriguing facts this way. For example, I learned about the lovely white aspen trees with their tinkling leaves. Aspen leaves quiver because of the special way the leaves are attached. They catch any little breeze. The sign describing these trees didn't say why that feature evolved. Does a quivering leaf have an evolutionary advantage over a more stationary one? Maybe it gives the leaf more chances at grabbing sunlight for photosynthesis. But that's just my theory. One of my theories. I invent theories all the time and wait for somebody else to do the tedious science.

The sign also conveyed the interesting fact that aspens seldom grow from seeds, like other trees do. Instead, they are said to be "clones," growing from the roots of other aspens. All the roots are interconnected underground. I don't know why they call that a clone, since it is still connected to its parent. It would seem to be more like one, huge, living organism, or at least like Siamese twins.

I stopped to look at a petrified tree. It looks like a tall tree stump, but it's rock. A couple of million years ago it got ashed during a volcanic eruption, and that preserved its form. It is guarded by a fence made of thick iron bars because its companion petrified tree got decimated by souvenir hunters. I said to the woman beside me, "A caged tree." She nodded and said, "A caged, petrified tree." Okay, not the high point of the trip.

I remembered seeing a petrified human at Pompeii where an eruption of Mt. Vesuvius encased an entire city in ash. I also watched from my living room window in awe as Mt. Saint Helens erupted in 1980, ashing everything in a thirty mile swath. I think it would be a privilege to be petrified in a volcanic eruption so that some future sentient being could say, "That's what Connie Crooker looked like two million years ago."

I went to tour Yellowstone's Norris Geyser Basin, but it was well into the afternoon, and I drooped. I'd been taking numerous short walks in the heat, I was somewhat oxygen deprived at this altitude, and I'd gotten sun exposure, although I'm super careful with hat and sunblock. The only reason I didn't get discouraged was that I felt so much better than I had two months prior, when I was still taking two-hour daily naps. I chose a handicapped parking space (yes, I've got that blue and white placard), and I took the shortest route into the basin to save steps.

At Norris, a chalky-white and sickly-yellow field, punctuated by steaming geysers and churning cauldrons of boiling water, spreads across the landscape. Wooden walkways allow you to wander there, inches above the steaming inferno that stinks like rotten eggs, convincing you that this place was not designed for humans. The signs emphasize the dangers from suddenly changing conditions in the geysers and fumaroles. Stepping off the walkway could mean falling into a boiling pit. There have been deaths, they warn you.

Getting splashed with the spray from a geyser made me jumpy. I had been reading how anything that hangs around these hot springs gets calcified over time from the constant spray. If you don't get petrified by a volcano, you can get calcified by a geyser. So many ways to go.

In spite of the hostile environment, there are living beings called thermophiles that love this place. In fact, they are so specialized that they can't live anyplace else. They feed off poisonous gases and they love scorching heat. Scientists are only beginning to learn about them. They are not life as we know it. They are life as we are stunned to discover it.

Scientists are just now discovering all kinds of "extremophiles" that live in conditions they thought could not support life. Some live in ice and some eat rust and some love totally dark caves. Knowing that life can adapt to harsh conditions means that the possibility of life elsewhere in the universe is increased. If life doesn't always require the moderate temperature range that we prefer, nor the atmosphere we require, then it could pop up anyplace. These thermophiles love to suck on sulfur that would gag a maggot. Who knew?

Scientists are only beginning to learn another thing. Almost the entire park is the crater of an ancient volcano. One volcano. Almost the whole park. We're talking big volcano. This was discovered only after satellites could photograph Yellowstone from high in orbit. The mountains that circle the park are the rim of an ancient crater, and the flat, smooth center of the park is the crater.

They call this a super volcano because it is so much more massive than Saint Helens or Vesuvius or others we know of. Scientists know it has erupted three times over the last several million years. Most recently it erupted about 600,000 years ago. Life that was located anywhere from present day Texas to Oregon would have perished in the massive blast.

Guess what. That volcano is still down there. A ranger told me that the craters of the three eruptions of the super volcano are not all in the same place. The crust of the earth moves in a process called tectonic shift, meaning the crust of rock we live on shifts over the surface of the molten stuff below. The earth had time to shift between the three eruptions of the super volcano, so the craters, though near each other, are not in identical spots, even though the volcano beneath is supposedly still in the same place. So, if the volcano erupts again, it may not be at the identical spot at the core of Yellowstone, but it will be close by.

The U.S. Geological Survey answers the question, "When will Yellowstone erupt again?" by saying, "We don't know." But here's what I wonder. In Lolo Pass I learned that when the pressure on the earth is released after an ice age, the gases gurgle in the earth creating more volcanic activity. At Yellowstone I saw a picture showing where the ice covered the park during the last ice age, a mere 10,000 years ago. The ice piled up in the basin of the old volcanic crater. It piled up thousands of feet thick and put pressure on a spot that was already sitting close to molten stuff below. Then the ice melted and released that pressure. Since then, gases must have been free to build up pressure down there under the old crater. And the whole area is indeed a patchwork of hot springs, geysers and fumaroles. Is anybody but me catching this connection? Are we in for another kaboom that will wipe out most of the western states? I'm just asking.

After leaving Norris Geyser Basin, I saw a sign that said, "Roaring Mountain," so I stopped to see if it were true. It is.

The white-streaked hillside is pockmarked with fumaroles and they do, indeed, roar. That is, when you can hear them over the passing traffic. And when you can hear them over loudly idling engines of boorish tourists who can't be bothered to step outside their cars. I was bold enough to approach one couple and say, all cheerfully—no accusations, "If you turn off your engine you can hear the roaring." Sheesh. What's with some people?

That evening I cooked a nice meal of fried pork chops and broccoli on my single burner camp-stove and enjoyed the solitude of writing in my journal beside my campfire under a starlit sky.

During the night I heard squealing that sounded like a cross between a yipping coyote and a donkey braying. It's the time of year. In September the buck elks are horny and lonely. This racket goes by the elegant name of "trumpeting." It sounds more like an asthmatic cat in heat.

In the morning my neighbor Ben told me the elk walked right between our campsites. I thought I heard snuffling outside my tent, but I was too afraid to peek out because the reality of seeing large mammals near my flimsy tent might keep me awake with images of getting trampled. My neighbor had slept in his pickup bed under the stars, so he had seen the elk walk by.

Ben is a 24-year-old, recently discharged from a six-year stint in the Navy. He was taking advantage of his newfound freedom from regimentation to wander the country in his pick-up, with minimal gear. He was trained as a Navy Seal, but he kept busting up various body parts and having multiple surgeries. He expects he'll have to fight the Navy's inevitable denial of his disability claim. He's well aware that this is our country's usual form of thanks to our injured veterans.

He was not stationed in Iraq, "but we lobbed stuff into there." He saw lots of good shore leave in Thailand and other Asian spots. He enjoyed Japan and Hawaii.

Light dances in Ben's eyes when he talks about his love for nature. His goal for this camping trip is to reconnect with nature and with God. One of the first things he did after his discharge was to hightail it to one of his favorite hiking spots on Mt. Rainier, as he had long ago promised himself he would.

We bragged to each other about how we seemed to be the only real campers in the campground. All the others buffered themselves from nature with their monster R.V.'s and their mounds of stuff that chained them like slaves to their gear. Ben wins extra points for sleeping in the open under the stars.

I had been cooking breakfast as we chatted, and I could see that he was nibbling on cold rations, so I offered him some hot bacon. His eyes lit up like he'd seen filet mignon.

My tent stakes weren't staying put in the sandy soil due to the wind. Ben helped me tie down my tent with some of his trusty parachute cord.

We discussed self-defense. Ben has a permit to carry a concealed weapon. I have chosen to forego that option, but I did consider both sides. Having written a book called, *Gun Control and Gun Rights,* I'm familiar with all the arguments and issues. Since I don't carry a firearm, he recommended a good-sized knife for me. He posed with his, hands on hips and legs astride, showing how threatening a knife can look dangling in the hand of a supremely confident person. Yup. Scary. He said I should keep the knife in my tent "so if a bear is coming in the front you can cut your way out the back."

I told him the Reader's Digest version of my escape from the maw of the Grim Reaper. He was impressed. He attributes it to God's will. I loved his jubilant spirit and didn't dispute his theory.

There are competing theories about my unexpected reprieve. My mother's church in small-town New Hampshire claims credit for their prayers. I don't share their theology, but I was, nonetheless grateful when I heard they were praying for me. All those good thoughts from people who care about me boosted my spirits. My dance and yoga instructors say it was because I kept moving and exercising. My friends tell me it's my attitude–that I'm optimistic–that I'm tough–that I kicked cancer's ass. My doctors believe they stumbled on a curative combo of interleukin-2 and radiation.

It turns out that radiation not only fries cancer cells but also lowers the number of regulatory T-cells in the body. Regulatory T-cells guard healthy cells from being attacked by the immune system. Melanoma cells disguise themselves as healthy cells by sending a chemical signal to marshal the body's regulatory T-cells. The T-cells act as sentries to protect melanoma from the immune system. If you lower the number of regulatory T-cells, while massively boosting the immune system with interleukin-2, the immune system finds its way to the unguarded melanoma cells and attacks them. That's the brand new theory of my melanoma oncologists.

I have told people that, in spite of the church, the yoga teacher, friends, and doctors, that the reason for my recovery was my thriftiness. In April of 2009, I bought a pre-season, discounted ski pass for the following winter, and was obliged to keep living so it wouldn't go to waste.

There actually was a sudden turning point from decline to recovery that seems a bit uncanny to a non-believer like me. This was in the winter of 2009, after radiation, during what I refer to as The Dreary Days; when I spent entire days on the couch. I didn't know then that I would enjoy this good period of recovery. I thought, "What if I never feel any better than this"? The "this" was rock bottom. If the radiation didn't work, as the interleukin-2 alone had not, then I was well on my way down the bottomless hill. The doctors hadn't promised much benefit from the radiation—only a last-ditch effort to help me eat without a bypass tube. And even that was not guaranteed.

So, during The Dreary Days, I went to put something in the dishwasher and I whacked my shin on the open dishwasher door. It hurt. I grabbed my leg and hopped around on one foot, wincing in pain. Then I cried. Then I sobbed uncontrollably. I discovered I could not stop crying. I cried for close to half an hour.

I cried from the hurt leg, and I cried from exhaustion. I cried about my long struggle through hideous treatments. I had marched bravely through surgery, interleukin-2 treatments, radiation, and multiple blood transfusions. I had worked a full-time job as the Professional Cancer Patient, and had done it stoically, with as much humor and grace as I could muster. But now the treatments were over, and very likely, my life. My optimism failed me. I cried over my upcoming death. I mourned my own passing.

I had not had a good, long cry for ages. I let myself see this cry through, beginning to end. I dove deeply into my despair. I thought every thought I had pushed aside for so long. I pictured leaving friends and family and I thought of their loss. I imagined shedding the possessions that had seemed so important to accumulate. I thought, at least I had seen my niece, Elizabeth be born and grow up. My melanoma was first diagnosed in 1990, the year before she was born, and it occurred to me I had been keeping it at bay just to help my sister raise her. Now she was grown, and I would have to say good-bye.

I had finished my part as the Professional Cancer Patient. Whatever would happen would happen. I give up. I turn myself over to ... to whatever forces of nature hold me in their web. I can't control the outcome of these treatments. I surrender. "Thy will be done." Not mine. If it must be death, I'm ready.

The very next day I felt lighter and brighter. And I've been improving ever since. I turned a corner toward recovery, and haven't yet relapsed. I suspect there's something about complete surrender to our utter helplessness in this vast universe that can heal. People think it's the fight that counts. They talk about battling cancer. They congratulate me on my tough attitude. From what I've seen of the ballsy women in my cancer support group, if a tough attitude could cure cancer, none would have died. But some *have* died. And if melanoma catches up with me, do I chastise myself for not being tough enough? I don't think so.

So, from that day, I was done battling this disease. I believe it's important to work to stay in shape to help the immune system with the healing process. But I swear, the moment I unconditionally accepted whatever might befall me, that's when my healing began.

◇◇◇◇◇

Chapter Six

That morning in the campground in Yellowstone, my first sight, on poking my nose out of my tent, was of two birds going for the pine nuts inside the cones on the tree above my tent. They pecked and prodded at the gaps in the pine cones with professional efficiency. My handy dandy Rocky Mountain Birds pamphlet says they are Clark's Nutcrackers. Aptly named. Hey, guess what. I lived long enough to see birds outside my tent again. Incredible.

After enjoying my breakfast-time talk with neighbor Ben, I wandered off again to sightsee, with no particular plan other than stopping when I felt like stopping. Mammoth Hot Springs was first in line.

Right next to the road, a massive white mound rises up in tiers, like a colossal, lumpy birthday cake dripping with white frosting. Just don't lick the spoon.

I drove up the hill and entered the area from the top, to avoid tiring myself on the tempting looking series of steps that start at the base of the mound. In better days I would have loved the challenge of climbing all those stairs, and I felt a pang of sadness that I was missing out, but the view from the top was perfectly satisfying.

Even more than the Norris Geyser Basin, this area makes clear that life as we know it is not welcome here. Charred branches of dead trees reach up from the white expanse. Apparently this place was once hospitable to vegetation, but it has been overwhelmed by poisonous gases and intolerable heat. I asked a ranger how long those dead trees had been there. She wasn't sure, but said that they show as dead stumps in photographs from the 1930's, so it's been awhile since anything lush lived there.

But thermophiles thrive. The ranger said that scientists are studying the genetics of different thermophiles in different areas of the park to see what the relationships might be. Since thermophiles can live only in specialized environments, scientists puzzle over how they get from one set of hot springs to another. It's not as if they produce seeds that blow in the wind.

I later posed this question to a Yale-educated friend–the question of how thermophiles might travel. He answered in one word: subways. He's not a scientist. He's a guy who, like myself, invents theories and waits for scientists to do the boring legwork. I bet he's onto something. Subways.

Mammoth Hot Springs is an awe-inspiring sight, even if you have no interest in reading the interpretive signs about thermophiles. Pools boil and bubble, and mist rises, and geysers spurt, and steaming water runs down the terraced hillside, and the scope of it all is just, well, mammoth.

Thermophiles got me pondering the origins of life. I like to read books written by scientists for laypeople. I call them my "science for dummies" books. My questions are sometimes answered by these books and sometimes not. Here's one of my unanswered questions about the origins of life.

Scientists say all life is related. They can look into our DNA and estimate how many generations back we shared a common ancestor with, say, squid. So, picture a single family tree. At the root is one cell. It divides and makes two, and they divide ... etc., etc. The copies aren't always identical to the original and some of the altered copies work out better than others. Differences start to form, shaped by natural selection until you reach the branches of the tree where we and the zebras and the penguins hang out. All one big family, right? But that unitary family relationship can only be true if one of two things happened.

One: There was only one cell that changed from dumb matter to a pulsing organism able to reproduce itself. One cell once came to life, divided, and that led to all of the rest of the living creatures. That would make us all related.

Or, Two: Conditions were right in the primordial slime for some unknown number of cells to spring to life. But unfortunately for most of them, something happened to kill off all their progeny, and only the descendants of one of those cells made it. Then, again, all life would be related.

But, what if life can spring into existence whenever certain conditions are ripe? What if new thermophiles, for example, are being brewed up all the time from inert matter? Then all of life would not be part of the same family tree. I asked the ranger about this, but, for some reason, she thought I was veering off into theology, and her eyes glazed over. But I'm curious about this. Is there one lifeline or could there be multiple, unrelated lifelines? I want Carl Sagan (*Forgotten Ancestors*) to come back just long enough to clear this up.

It's an important question, because the answer would tell us whether the original animation of inanimate matter was a unique hiccup unlikely to reoccur, or whether it's a process repeatable under the right conditions. If it's repeatable, then the likelihood of life elsewhere in the universe is increased. I won't speculate on mad scientists creating ... never mind.

Of course there's a clash between scientists and some religious believers about the origins of life. I think we do a disservice to describe them as competing camps. Religion can't do what science does, and vice versa. They are not simply two different belief systems. Religion is a belief system and science is a process.

Science is a process of investigation that follows certain rules (embodied in the scientific method) that have proved to produce useful results. Science works well because it admits the possibility of being wrong. The error in any scientific theory can be corrected by any subsequent scientist who spots its flaws.

Religion, on the other hand, claims a pipeline to truth. It is not open to error. It's the Divine Word. So, there's no sense putting religion and science on the same scale to weigh truth. Religion is about spirit and our experience of it. People talk about it in allegories and parables. Since nobody can prove religious assertions, you are asked to take them on faith.

Science is about how stuff works, and relies on rigorous proof, repeatable by any scientist who runs the same test. Why would we expect the creation fables we have told over generations (serpents and gardens, or ravens and coyotes) to produce the same kinds of truth as a process that has come up with computers and rockets and interleukin-2? If you have questions about good and evil, see your pastor. If you have questions about how the world works, or how old it is, or how life evolved on it, talk to a scientist. Contrary to claims of self-styled "creationists," religion is not a science and science is not a religion. As the bumper sticker says, "Get your theology out of my biology."

At lunchtime, I followed signs to the Sheepeater Cliff picnic area. Fortunately, all the picnic tables were taken, forcing me to retreat to a more peaceful spot. I carried my sandwich to the riverbank where I took off my shoes and dangled my tootsies in the brisk, clear water of the Gardner River. I munched my lunch and enjoyed moments of solitude. It often takes only a small effort to get away from the teeming hordes. I even found a private spot to pee in the bushes. One of life's finer pleasures is squatting in the wild with a cool breeze to tickle your fanny.

Nothing much beats that feeling of freedom.

I found my way back to civilization—a store where I succumbed to ice cream and, yes, a souvenir. I'm no sucker for souvenirs, but I got waylaid by nostalgia. I remembered how, in 1959, I searched all the gift shops in the West before spending my hard-earned allowance on one special item, because that was all I could afford. In those days there was an abundance of cheap goldstone jewelry for sale everywhere. I loved the way the golden specks glinted in the caramel-brown stone. I lusted for a piece of goldstone jewelry. Finally I bought a goldstone bracelet. I remember that bracelet. I loved that bracelet. Sometimes a souvenir is more than a cheap bauble. It is what a souvenir is supposed to be; a memory. So this time I picked out an inexpensive necklace: a string of raw turquoise and obsidian. I love that necklace. I have been wearing it daily. It's my Yellowstone necklace, even if it was made in Taiwan.

That night, just after dark, light flashed in the sky to the north. Then again to the northwest. Then the west. Then southwest. Earth jarring, explosive sounds accompanied the light show. I knew by the way it moved across the sky that it must be a thunderstorm, but my worries about the explosive, volcanic powder keg I was sitting on made me twitchy.

I thought, how quickly should I prepare for the storm? Sometimes in the desert you watch a storm pass in a line over there and it never gets over here. I didn't have long to wonder. The rain started in single, cold plops, then turned into a steady drizzle.

I make it a rule not to sleep in a tent during a thunderstorm. It's safer in a car that gives some protection from falling trees. This is not theoretical.

During a prior trip, while camping in Ohio I had bedded down in my tent in fine weather when a violent thunderstorm struck. I considered switching my bedding to the relative safety of the car, but it rained so hard I chose not to risk getting drenched and chilled, so I stayed put. The storm kept on throughout the night. I would drift to sleep only to be awakened repeatedly by heart-stopping crashes, rolls, and rumbles. One crash was so loud and so close by that I acutely felt my vulnerability to raging nature. I was not one of your proverbial happy campers.

In the morning I crawled out of my soggy tent to behold an enormous tree on its side in the campsite two spaces down from mine. Lightening had struck it, and that tree was a goner. Thankfully the site was empty of campers. If I had chosen that spot I would have been mashed to hamburger, if I hadn't been fried first by lightning. So that's why I don't stay in a tent during a thunderstorm.

With the storm approaching the campground in Yellowstone, I needed to make a plan. The back seat of my car was already down flat, so there was room for me to sleep there. First I donned my rain poncho. Getting wet and chilled in the outdoors is never a good idea. Then I rapidly piled all my gear on one side of the car and put my bedding down on the other. My air mattress was too wide for the narrow space, so the bed wasn't soft, but I would have to make do.

The wind kicked up and blew my tent into the oddest shapes, like twisted parabolas and Moebius strips. Only Ben's parachute cord kept it from blowing away, but the twisting motions were warping the tent poles. I was afraid they would break, so I collapsed the tent and piled firewood on it to hold it in place.

I snuggled into my bed in the car and watched the dramatic flashes from the storm. As it turns out, the storm soon passed. But I was not convinced. The stars hadn't yet returned, and the clouds could open up at any time, so I watched and waited. After more than an hour with no lightening or thunder, I longed for my comfortable tent, but it was late and I was tired. It would take time to set up my tent, blow up my air mattress, and move my gear again. I tried to drift off to sleep in the car, but couldn't convince myself that the cramped quarters and the hard floor were cozy. I needed my nice little bed.

I finally got up and reversed the entire process. Firewood off the tent, tent shaken out to get the rain off, tent pitched again in darkness, air mattress pumped up, sleeping bag moved from car to tent, red Folger's coffee can in its place. I crawled into my warm, dry sleeping bag. I checked my travel alarm clock. Midnight. I patted myself on the back. I thought, look at me. Aren't I something. I can handle whatever nature throws at me. I feel good about camping. I like camping. I like my comfy bed and my fluffy, warm sleeping bag pulled up to my neck. Good night, world.

In the morning, while I was enjoying some leisurely puttering around my campsite, I witnessed The Invasion of The Elk. Females were filtering down the hill through sparse trees toward the campground. A male was trumpeting his by-now-familiar call. His high pitched whining sounded so forlorn that even I was tempted to offer the poor guy a mercy fuck. Then he appeared, following the females with his full rack of antlers bobbing and swaying. Elk are massive creatures. Although they are in the deer family, they lack the deer's dainty, slender grace. They are deer on steroids.

People in their R.V.'s actually stepped outside to watch the elk show. Watch out, folks. There's fresh air out here.

The ranger came around in his ranger van and stayed close to the elk. The ranger had a heck of a job keeping the *homo sapiens* from mingling with the *cervus canadensis*. When elk get horny, they are moody and unpredictable. They are not pets.

This male wasn't interested in charging any people, because he found another male elk to charge. He wandered across the street below the campground and into an open field right next to the road where all the cars could easily stop to watch him. I think he was on the payroll of the Discovery Channel.

The two males looked equally matched from my vantage point. They lowered their heads and came at each other, locking antlers and clashing with a marvelously resonant clacking and clattering like syncopated drumbeats of the wild. They pawed and dug at the dry soil with their hooves, raising clouds of brown dust. They circled and snorted and clashed for more than half an hour.

In the campsite across from mine was a darling Korean-American boy, no more than four years old, who got excited by the fray. He put his hands up by his head to make antlers, and he snorted and pawed the ground with his little foot while charging his invisible foe. Testosterone poisoning knows no bounds.

A ranger told me that the elk were trying to gouge each other's throats, but if they failed at that, they would fight until one got exhausted. That's exactly what happened. One of them finally disengaged, turned and ran off, rapidly at first, as if to escape, then at a slow trot. The other ambled along behind him, probably monitoring his departure, to make sure he didn't sneak around in the bushes to return for a quickie with the girls.

I was interested in the reaction of the females during all this. There was very little reaction. They kept happily munching on leaves while minding their young ones, pretty much ignoring the ruckus. Every once in a while, a loud male snort would cause them to raise their heads, but I don't think they cared which imperious bully prevailed. Either winner would boss them around, herding them here and there.

Speaking of munching on leaves, several of the females discovered that some leaves in my campsite, right beside my tent, were tasty. There's a park rule that you are supposed to stay twenty-five yards from the animals, but they forgot to inform the elk. They were all crowding in on me, so I backed up to the other side of my car to let them snack away. But when one of the youngsters decided to taste my tent, I found myself approaching and saying, "Shoo, little elk. Shoo." I wonder if the tent tasted salty from waterproofing spray, or if young elk, like human children, will put just anything in their mouths.

After The Invasion of The Elk it was time to pack up my gear and head out for my leisurely drive out of the park.

◇◇◇◇◇

Chapter Seven

While driving down the road, I have time to ponder, soliloquize, and imagine the world as a better place. I found my notes for these thoughts on medical care in my travel journal, and will share them here.

In my dealings with the medical world, I have noticed that patients have varied attitudes toward doctors. Consumers of medical services seem to fall into one of three camps: the overly trusting, the overly skeptical, and those who participate in their own health care.

The first group consists of those who unquestioningly trust the whole system: their doctors, pharmacists, and even, heaven help them, their health insurance companies. They find it easier to follow marching orders than to ask questions. This is understandable. When you are sick, you need to feel you can rely on others, and you lack the energy to cross-examine your doctors. The docs have the training, and you don't. Might as well do what they say. But busy medical professionals can miss important facts or fail to communicate well with a complex team of service providers, and things do fall through the cracks. It never hurts to double check their orders. It also helps to have a friend or family member advocate for you when your own fighting spirit has abandoned you.

The second group distrusts what they call "the medical establishment." They see one big conspiracy to pocket their money at the expense of their health. Most any "alternative" treatment seems more alluring to them than standard medical care. But by avoiding being suckered by "big business," they fail to see how they are being suckered by quacks and snake oil salesmen.

I once got an email from a friend of a friend who had heard about my recovery. She wanted reassurance that she was right to forego chemotherapy for a highly touted alternative drug. She complained that chemotherapy was too harsh, and she wanted a gentler treatment. Although I don't give unsolicited advice about medical care, she had asked, so I checked the American Cancer Society's website and quickly learned that her chosen treatment had a track record of zero for curing cancer. I sent her a link to the site and told her, while the elderly and infirm may reasonably forego the rigors of chemotherapy, that cancer is not gentle with you, so why should you be gentle with it? I wish this woman well, but worry that she might have made a deadly mistake by relying on the kinder-gentler-cancer-cure claims of some practitioners of alternative medicine.

Not that mainstream practitioners don't offer alternative treatments. They do. They come in the form of clinical trials. I was ready to participate in several, but didn't meet their parameters for various reasons. But for somebody, like me, who has been told that I'm likely to die with standard care alone, a clinical trial can offer both standard care and alternative care. Doctors who offer clinical trials are not averse to trying something new when all else has failed.

Here's how clinical trials generally work. With your informed consent, they give you standard care such as chemo. They also give you the new product or procedure they are studying, or they might give you a placebo. They run the study on a number of patients and compare results. You are warned that the new treatment may not work or that you may have been randomly selected to receive the placebo. This is science, and it is not unethical, since you are getting the standard care they would have given you anyway.

I lean toward science-based medicine because it compares

people who get the treatment with people who don't, and can tell us how likely it is that a treatment will work for us. Other systems rely on what science calls "anecdotal evidence."

Here's an example of the difference. Your Uncle Ed is a lifelong smoker and he lives to the ripe old age of 100 with no lung cancer, so you conclude that smoking does not lead to lung cancer. That's "anecdotal evidence" based on observation of one case. But Uncle Ed could be the exception to the rule.

Science would take, say, a thousand smokers and a thousand non-smokers and compare their incidence of lung cancer. If the smokers show more lung cancer, the scientists would ask themselves, how much more? Is the difference big enough to be "statistically significant?" If so, scientists can say that smokers have more lung cancer *because* of the smoking.

Suzanne Somers has written a controversial book called *Knockout* in which she promotes alternative cancer treatments over those approved by the medical establishment. Her book has been criticized for not distinguishing between claims based on anecdotal evidence and those based on properly conducted scientific studies. This matters because she is an influential popular personality, and if she turns out to be wrong, her advice could kill. Here's what Dr. Otis Brawley, chief medical officer of the American Cancer Society has said about her: "I am very afraid that people are going to listen to her message and follow what she says and be harmed by it. We use current treatments because they've been proven to prolong life. They've gone through a logical scientific method of evaluation. I don't know if Suzanne Somers even knows there IS a logical, scientific method."

Many of those who are skeptical of the medical establishment, including Suzanne Somers, claim that the medical establishment's greed trumps their goal of curing us. I haven't experienced that. My melanoma oncologists, Dr. Ernstoff at Dartmouth-Hitchcock in New Hampshire, and Dr. Curti at Providence in Oregon, are both brainy, curious guys with lots of heart. They're out to cure melanoma and they're rooting for my immune system just as I am. They're delighted to see me alive and happy. So don't knock your doc unless your doc is a dope.

The third group of medical consumers participates in their own health care. One way is to write out questions before doctor's appointments and to take notes during the appointments. I don't let my doctors rush to the next patient until I've double checked my list of questions. If an appointment deals with a major decision, I ask a family member to participate. This is especially important when I'm feeling so sick that I can't absorb all the information.

This group of medical consumers relies on standard medical care, but may use wisdom that comes from outside standard regimens to supplement their care. For example, it is known that there are health benefits from massage therapy, good diet, yoga, meditation, and even prayer. These things may boost the immune system, which aids healing, or, at the very least, may improve the quality of life of the dying person. Although there's danger in using these practices as a substitute for standard care, they can enhance it.

The oft-maligned medical establishment is beginning to recognize the importance of alternative systems as aids in healing. For example, Providence Hospital in Portland, Oregon offers massage therapy and acupuncture to supplement standard treatments. Many hospitals provide chapels for prayer and meditation.

Providence Hospital also offers a free, weekly support group for women with late-stage cancer. It is called, *Making Today Count*. I have participated for several years, and find it immensely helpful. We women talk frankly about our medical treatments and our fears of dying. As the group's name suggests, we share tips on making the most of our days, even when they are few. We "pass the candle" in memory of a group member who dies. We drop the brave public front and we cry with others who understand our ordeals, that is, when we aren't howling with laughter. Participating in the support group makes us feel better, which likely boosts our immune systems. But these down-to-earth gab fests are not intended as a cure. Many of us die. The support group helps ease the process, whichever way it goes.

These are the kinds of thoughts I have time to ponder while driving down the road.

On my way out of the park I stopped at the large and lovely Yellowstone Lake. It was a windy day, and the lake was dotted with white caps and framed by distant mountains. In 1959, we had camped near the lakeshore. I stood and gazed across the lake, trying to remember where it was that I had played kissy-face in the bushes with Neal.

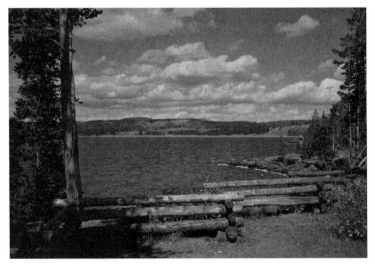

Back in our Ozzie and Harriet days, while driving across Wyoming towards Yellowstone, our sky-blue Plymouth played hopscotch with a VW bug. There were two cute guys in the bug. The driver caught big sister Carol's eye. The young boy, Neal, with curly, sun-streaked hair, and creamy, golden skin, caught mine. My family went to a rodeo in Cody, Wyoming, and these two cute guys from the VW show up. We chat. We flirt. We wish our parents would evaporate.

We bump into the boys a couple more times along the way, and then, in the campground by Lake Yellowstone, there they are, setting up a newfangled, nylon dome tent. It was the first time I'd seen one, and I was impressed with how quickly they assembled it. It was much like the one I use now. Back then, our family's tents were the cumbersome canvas style, likely left over from the Lewis and Clark expedition.

We find out there's a dance in the park. The cute guys invite Carol and me to go. I don't remember if we planted the idea, as girls often do, or if they surprised us. What I remember is hunkering down in the bushes by the lake with Neal so we could practice our kissing. At age 12, I was not in love. I was taking advantage of an opportunity to build lipwork skills for future reference. Come to think of it, I was using the guy. Neal was a couple of years older than I, but still a kid himself. I sensed he wanted to pour extra ardor into the endeavor, but in the 1950's we girls knew where the line was. Nothing below the neck, Neal. That's a no-no. Not that I had anything below the neck worth exploring.

Only a few years ago my sister Carol was taking a cruise on a boat on a New Hampshire lake, and she noticed the name of the captain. It was the driver of the VW. They chatted and reminisced about Yellowstone and the dance. Carol learned that the fellow had been acting as Big Brother to Neal, who was a troubled kid from the projects. That didn't surprise me one bit. I've got a built-in magnet for the bad boys.

Back to the glorious trip. I wanted to spend more time by Yellowstone Lake, so I checked my map for a picnic area. When I got there, the wind was whipping across the lake and chilling down an otherwise sunny day. Instead of attempting to construct a sandwich in the maelstrom, I munched a few salty snacks and accidentally-on-purpose dropped one to see if the parking lot raven-in-residence would come close enough to snatch it. Yeah, yeah, yeah. I know not to feed the wildlife. They get dependent on us. Our food isn't healthy for them. It's not good for them to lose their fear of people. But I do make an occasional exception for parking lot ravens. I figure it this way.

Ravens are smart enough to benefit from hanging around the rich folk. That'd be us. It's tough to make it in the wilderness. We humans are famous for wiping out entire species, but sometimes our rich lifestyle benefits wildlife. For example, I see fewer hawks in the wilderness than I do near farmers' fields. The crops attract rodents and the rodents attract hawks. If the rodents haven't been poisoned with pesticides, the hawks benefit from our agriculture. The same goes for seagulls. They follow fishermen and snatch fish guts and half-eaten Snickers bars. Seagulls are abundant in seaports and scarce on isolated beaches.

Ravens are bold enough to claim leftovers from our picnics. Our food may not nourish them, but it does have salt, which is scarce in the wild. Birds need some salt. Polly want a cracker. So I dropped a salty snack, and my new friend danced and bobbed nearby, but wouldn't come close enough to snatch it until he saw competition approaching. The second raven puffed out his chest and began goose-stepping toward the morsel with a confident waddle. The first one scurried past him, grabbed the snack in his beak, and retreated to a safe distance.

People say that feeding wild birds makes them dependent on humans. Won't the raven starve in the winter when the tourists leave? I doubt it. What do birds do when the berries on the bushes dry up? They fly away and find food elsewhere. They're not chained to the parking lot. And these are very smart birds. But you really shouldn't feed them. I'm just justifying my bad behavior.

I drove down, down, down a steep canyon toward the east entrance to the park. There are dramatic views and the thrill of perching on the side of potentially unstable geology. The sudden drop in elevation makes sense when you consider that you have left a volcanic crater and are driving to the base of an old, old mountain.

After leaving Yellowstone, the scenery takes a dramatic turn toward cowboy-movie-backdrop with pillars of layered rocks in reddish-brown hues, and with desert-like land. I got drowsy by mid-afternoon, so I pulled into a lovely picnic area where a trout stream gurgles and trees rustle and cicadas buzz and click. A couple came up from the stream carrying two good-sized fish, still wet and glistening. When they drove off, I had the place to myself.

I unfolded my camp chair into a flat cot, grabbed my pillow and took the most luscious nap in the shade, with a cool breeze tickling my happy nose. This was the most peaceful moment yet of my trip. Yellowstone is a thrill-a-minute place, bustling with humanoid life forms, but here, by the river, the sunny, peaceful world was mine, all mine.

As I headed east, the landscape flattened out into ranchland. I arrived at Cody, Wyoming, scene of the 1959 flirtation with the cute boys at the rodeo. This time I was only passing through. I spotted a Sierra Trading Post outlet store. They sell discounted outdoor gear, and I'm a sucker for a bargain. I stopped to look for a knife, because Ben's suggestion about self-defense made sense to me. They had an array of tempting knives that would last for generations, but I figured that carving my way out of the back of the tent as the bear enters the front would be a one-time event, and wouldn't require durability, so I chose the five-buck model.

I passed through the smaller city of Greybull, Wyoming, which has a county airport with a giant "In God We Trust" painted on the side of one of its buildings. The airport is strewn with carcasses of military planes. The planes are apparently repaired there, but it looks more like a U-Pull-It car lot, except that it's our tax dollars rusting away. Anybody for a used stealth fighter jet?

Greybull also has a huge facility for mining bentonite. I had to look up that one. Bentonite is a kind of muddy clay that is formed when volcanic ash gets wet. I bet we know where all that volcanic ash came from. Greybull is not all that far from Yellowstone. Kaboom!

So how has human ingenuity come up with a way to market wet volcanic ash? Here is a list of its uses from the Wyo-Ben company: "oil, gas, and water well drilling, metalcasting, environmental construction and remediation, hazardous waste treatment, cat litter, cosmetics and pharmaceuticals, as well as many other industrial and consumer related products." Cosmetics? "I'll have the volcanic mud facial, please."

I drove through Wyoming's Bighorn Mountains late in the afternoon. I instantly fell in love and could have kicked myself for not carving out more time to explore its bare naked geology. But the drive had drama because of the late time of day and the lateness in the season. My lovely string of 80-degree days had ended. It was cold up there.

The road winds up rocky ravines that display all the workings of the earth in past geological eras. Roadside signs point to different layers in the cliffs and tell how many hundreds of millions of years ago those rocks formed. If you know your geology, it's like looking at time lapse photography of the earth's changes, most of which happened before humans evolved. Humanity's brief sojourn on the planet has been a passing fancy in time's kaleidoscope. We think we're hot stuff, but we're blind to our insignificance.

We're an aggressive species puffed up with self-importance. We're voraciously acquisitive, overabundant, gratuitously violent, and, ever since we migrated off the African continent, we have functioned as an invasive species everywhere we've trampled, supplanting entire ecosystems in our wake. But still we have our charms. We can be clever, curious, and even cuddly.

The same characteristic that causes us to wreak so much havoc might be our saving grace: our smarts. We are not merely smart and clever. We are conscious to an uncanny degree. I suspect that the nature of our consciousness might be unique. Many animals are smart enough to solve survival problems, but I doubt that other animals wonder about how big the universe is, and what happens after they die, and who will be the next American Idol.

I was once in a discussion group where we talked about the nature of our humanity. One of the members was the actor, Chuck Gray, who used to play cowboy roles on black-and-white television shows. He sat quietly in a corner, and only contributed one idea, but it was memorable. He said, "We're here so the universe can be conscious of itself."

We're carbon-based bits of stardust, animated and awake. We gaze into the universe and see all the burning, freezing, exploding, and gravity-sucking hazards out there. It's all hostile to our frail existence inside this thin layer of oxygen on the barely cooled-off surface of this smallish planet. Yet our brains can reach back to calculate the beginnings of time and space, and we know how fast light travels, and we know what the red shift tells us about how far away the stars are. That expansiveness of thought is a special kind of consciousness. Perhaps we *are* here so the universe can be conscious of itself.

I'm always thinking about the speed of light. I'm not kidding. When you lack a boyfriend, you have to worry about something, so I noodle over the speed of light. It was Einstein who shocked us with the news that our watches run at different speeds depending on how fast we're moving relative to each other.

Say you've got this train whizzing along at half the speed of light, and you've got Romeo standing on the platform watching the train, and Juliet sitting on the train with a photon clock on the floor beside her. Think of a photon as a teensy particle of light. Scientists tell us that a photon always moves at the speed of light, which is fast. The speed of light is our cosmic speed limit; nothing in the universe can travel faster than the speed of light. Juliet's clock consists of one photon that begins its journey at the train's floor and travels eight feet to the ceiling, then back another eight feet to the floor. Tick tock. From Juliet's perspective her photon clock marks out sixteen feet at the speed of light.

No way, says Romeo who stands on the platform watching the train whizz past. For that photon to travel to the ceiling and back to the floor, it must travel much farther than sixteen feet because, after it leaves the floor, and before it bounces off the ceiling, the ceiling of the speeding train has moved way off down the line. It has moved so far away that the photon has to move on a big, long diagonal that is much longer than eight feet. Picture two long diagonal lines, one going up to the now distant ceiling, and the other coming back down to meet the floor which has moved even farther down the line. Because of our cosmic speed limit, the photon can only move at the speed of light. So from Romeo's vantage point, it takes longer for that first tick tock than from Juliet's point of view, because the distance the photon must travel is longer, and the photon can't travel any faster.

Now suppose the speeding train circles back to where Romeo stands on the platform. Juliet, still seated on the moving train, checks her photon clock and sees that maybe about an hour has passed. So who's that old geezer on the platform looking like Romeo's great grandfather? That's right. It's a decrepit Romeo who sees a hot young babe on the train, and wonders why she looks so familiar.

The relativity of time has been proven by scientists who sent a real and exceedingly accurate atomic clock on a spacecraft that moved pretty darn fast. When it got back to earth the clock showed that less time had passed than our earth clocks had measured. This is because, to the earth observer of a speeding object, each tick tock takes longer than a tick tock takes on the speeding object itself. Thus, the clock that went into space returned showing that less time had passed.

Push it one more step. Now the train's going at the speed of light. From Romeo's point of view, the diagonals get so stretched out they are no longer diagonal. They flatline. Time gets all used up. No more tick tock. The photon sits on the floor in a state of surprised expectation, waiting to start its upward journey to mark the progress in Juliet's day, but there is no progress. The train's motion at the speed of light superglues the photon to the floor and it's not budging. The train's moving so fast the photon can't lift off the floor because it's using all its allowable speed to travel sideways with the train at the speed of light.

Nothing can break the cosmic speed limit, so, at the speed of light, there's no tick tock. Time stands still. If a conscious being could travel at the speed of light, that's how time would seem. Simply vanished. No past. No future.

What can that possibly mean? We are said to live in a four-dimensional universe: three spatial dimensions and one dimension of time. If you chit-chat with a string theorist, the spacial dimensions start multiplying, but the principle is the same. We've got only space and time to work with. That's the whole show, universe-wise.

So if the photon uses up all its time because it's traveling at the speed of light, which photons always do, then what would a self-aware photon perceive about space? Romeo sees a photon leave the sun and take eight minutes to travel to earth. But to a photon, because it always travels at the speed of light, no time has passed. It doesn't say, "I used to be at the sun and in a few minutes I'm going to be on earth." It has no past or future. So the earth and the sun must seem all the same to the photon. It must be located everywhere it's ever been and everywhere it will ever be, all at once. It must be hanging perpetually in some glowing god time–a kind of noplace or everyplace–a Buddha-like oneness that brims with light and energy.

If we define the universe as a combination of space and time, and yet something as ordinary as light experiences neither, somebody has some 'splaining to do.

Here's something else weird about photons. They are capable of what Einstein called spooky action at a distance, and what scientists now call entanglement. What exactly entangled photons are you can ask the hot-shots, but picture what used to be one photon becoming two photons. Photon clones more or less. If you fiddle with one of them over here, the other acts identically, in complete synch with the first, no matter how far away it is. And it does so instantaneously. It's not waiting for the first photon to send it information at the speed of light telling it how to behave.

How can these photons dance in perfect synch if they don't have time to send each other messages across space? Scientists are still scratching their heads over this one, even when they observe it right under their noses.

I'm guessing here, but I wonder if it has something to do with photons not existing in time and space in the same way that we do. We know they don't experience time, because they always move at the speed of light. What if, from their point of view, they're not separated in space? If time is always now and space is always here, and the entangled photons were once together, then maybe there's never any distance between them.

So our self-aware particle of light might see itself as just a pulsing glowing stillness—a throbbing godlike calm at the heart of things, pumping power into the system. This would come as no surprise to the ancient Mayans or Druids or any of the sun worshipers who have marveled at the awesome gift and treacherous danger of sunshine. Of course light's a god. Who could doubt it?

◇◇◇◇◇

Chapter Eight

As I drove up past the rocky area of the Bighorns, I reached high altitude meadows where cattle grazed on the open range. In one herd I saw, out of the corner of my eye, an animal that was the wrong shape. I looked again. It was a "lang-leggedy" moose ambling right through the herd. This car brakes for wildlife. I pulled over and watched.

The moose seemed oblivious to the cattle. He wandered through as if he didn't see them, which might have been true. My mother taught me that when I come upon a moose in the wild I should hide behind a tree because they have bad eyesight and can't see you there. But this moose caught sight of one of its bovine companions. And vice versa. Uh oh. Two steps forward by the moose. Two steps forward by the steer. Hides go all twitchy and the moose drools. The moose surveys its foe. It rules out a wolf that might bite its flank. It rules out another moose that will charge it. Oh yeah. A dumb domesticated beast. No problem. The moose turns and ambles off, leaving its exposed hindquarters wide open.

The pass at the top of the Bighorns is a whopping 9,000 feet above sea level. I've climbed difficult mountains half that high. When I passed through on this late September afternoon, the sky was a thick and darkening grey. Streaks of white began blowing sideways across the open landscape. Snow. The snowfall thickened and blocked the view of the surrounding mountains. Soon, all I saw was a white, sideways blur with a dark grey backdrop. At least I could see the road, which I hoped would not turn icy. I clutched the steering wheel tight in case of a skid. I twisted down that mountain road, staying alert to trouble. It was white knuckle driving, but I felt the thrill of adventure, because the storm was so dramatic, and I was so alone and exposed. Fortunately, I was on its front edge, and I made it safely down to Sheridan, Wyoming just in time. The next morning, three inches of gleaming snow graced the lovely Bighorns.

I had telephoned a reservation to a campground in Sheridan, but arrived after dark, to discover that it was cold and raining. The wind howled and churned with a tent-threatening fury. I'll camp in cold, or in rain, or in wind, but I'll skip the triple-play combo, thank you. The campground managers directed me to a locally-owned motel, the Trail's End, which was decorated in vintage Cowboy and Indian, and which included a trucker-approved buffet breakfast with the modest price of the room. I wrote in my log, "First shower since Gardiner. Three days? Four? I lost track." And you wonder why I have no boyfriend.

The next morning, just outside of Sheridan, I began to see herds of pronghorn antelope. They are easy to distinguish from deer because antelope have white patches on each side, and big, white rumps. Their short antlers curve inwards and only have a single prong for an offshoot, not a full rack like a deer's. One antelope was running with stately grace across the plains. They are thought to be the fastest mammal in North America. Their speed may have evolved to outrun catlike predators that are now extinct, because they can run faster than is necessary to escape today's wolves and cougars. "Oh give me a home where the buffalo roam, and the deer and the antelope play, where seldom is heard a discouraging word, and the sky is not cloudy all day." Does that mean the sky is only cloudy for some of the day, or that it is sunny all day? I stew over such things.

I drove through rolling ranchland, which, as I got farther east, was broken up by rocks that appeared to have been exposed by erosion—like badlands in their infancy. An interpretive sign at a rest area explained the Texas Trail, which had passed through the area. It was a twenty-mile-wide network of cattle trails used for driving cattle north from Texas during the late 1800's. The sign said that the trail's purpose was to replace the waning buffalo and "bring civilization to the West." It honest-to-god said that. I wonder what all those savage Indians would think of that. You know, the primitive creatures who welcomed Lewis and Clark with food and friendship instead of scalping them.

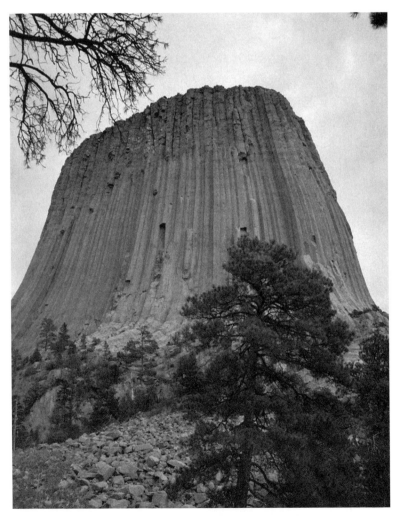

Speaking of Indians, I visited Devils Tower (the white-man's name), which is a sacred site to many Indian tribes. Their name for it usually involves a bear, in whatever tribal language, because they say it was formed by a giant bear clawing its sides to try to reach some kids who were hiding on top. Geologists say it is a volcanic plug that formed hexagonal granite pillars as it cooled. The evenness of the symmetry of the huge pillars is striking.

A ranger told me that our name, Devils Tower may have come from a misunderstanding of the pronunciation of one of the Indian tribes' bear names——we thought they said "evil doer" instead of bear. I suggested that perhaps when the pious settlers saw a pack of heathens worshiping a rock, they excoriated those red devils. Thus, Devils Tower. The ranger admitted I might have something there.

Rock climbers love the challenge of climbing the vertical walls of Devils Tower. Indians hate to see white guys crawl all over their sacred site. The controversy has been long and serious enough that the Indians convinced the Forest Service to declare the month of June as a time of Indian pilgrimage to the site. The Forest Service recommends that climbers voluntarily refrain from climbing during that month. Most do, but a few climbers took their case to court, asking the federal court to declare the Forest Service in violation of the First Amendment (which mandates separation of church and state) for involving itself in support of Indian religious practices. The Tenth Circuit Court of Appeals ducked the issue by telling the hikers that they had no standing to sue since they were not injured by the alleged violation. The Forest Service was merely making a suggestion; the climbers could climb the rock any time they felt like it. No harm, no foul. End of lawsuit.

I admit to mixed feelings about respecting the Indians'

spiritual practices simply because I wonder about the wisdom of kowtowing to anybody's religious mythology. I feel a bit patronizing when I nod and smile at spiritual hocus pocus while secretly thinking, "These kids still believe in Santa." Maybe I should say what I'm really thinking; "You believe what? Are you shittin' me?" I'm talking about all religions. I'm an equal opportunity skeptic. A virgin gave birth to a god. Come again? A snake handed a woman an apple, and when she took a bite, she fell asleep until a prince kissed her. Or am I mixing things up?

My skepticism aside, it makes sense to me why the Indians are as aghast at climbers on their temple as some of us would be at seeing climbers on Notre Dame Cathedral. But really, wouldn't it be fun to climb Notre Dame? The Indians should organize a Notre Dame climbing party led by Quasimodo.

At the visitors center, I saw a man in the parking lot who had arrived in a gleaming, canary-yellow, '55 Chevy convertible. Perfection on wheels. When I see a '55 Chevy, I hear Fats Domino singing *Blueberry Hill.* I see us girls wearing bobby sox and circular skirts that are poofed out with two or three stacked, crinoline petticoats. I taste root beer floats. I had seen the same car in Yellowstone the day before and I had waxed nostalgic. This time I went up to the man and told him his car reminded me of our 1956, sky-blue Plymouth station wagon that we drove to Yellowstone in the fifties. I said that I've often wondered if anybody restored it, or if it had become a pancake of scrap metal. He said, "It's probably a Toyota now."

Back to our hunka hunka rock. I almost didn't stop here because it was a bit out of the way, and who wants to see a solitary rock when the West is riddled with rocks. But I made the extra effort because of my America the Beautiful pass. Devils Tower is a national monument, and my pass would get me free admission. Can't miss that deal.

As soon as I saw Devils Tower, I was hooked. It inspires awe for its singular beauty, with its top-to-bottom hexagonal granite pillars stacked together like sheaves of wheat. It is a looming, imposing presence, not to be ignored. It draws you in. Combine that with its solitary locale–no nearby drama queens to distract us–and we've got a rock worth venerating. Birds nest in its crevices, climbers scramble over it, and Indians leave their medicine bundles tied to trees beside it.

The clusters of colorful, cloth medicine bundles reminded me of clootie rags in Scotland. I once saw a spring there that was famous amongst the locals for its healing properties. For generations the sick brought fabric items that had touched their bodies–handkerchiefs, scarves, or just plain rags–and they dipped the cloths in the healing waters and tied them to a nearby bush while praying for health. This had been going on for so long that clootie rags on top of clootie rags faded and rotted in the open air. It was an unsightly mess. The town fathers offered to pay to have them removed, but could find nobody willing to do it. Too much spirit stuff going on there.

Of course, I wouldn't be so superstitious. Not science-minded me. But when I was in the depths of despair from my hideous interleukin-2 treatments, I developed a daily ritual that might come as a surprise. I have an African rattle——a crude thing made from a hollowed-out gourd perched on a jagged stick. When I shake it, the seeds inside make a rich, tinkling sound. I used to lie down and shake the rattle directly above the inoperable tumor in my chest. I would relax so that I could feel the rattle's vibrations in my chest. I would focus on the tightness and the pain and try to rattle it loose. I would tell my tumor it was free to leave me now. Tumor, I don't need you. You can go now. Rattle, rattle, rattle. Goodbye, tumor. Rattle, rattle,

rattle. With this daily ritual I could relax a bit and my deep terror would temporarily subside.

This from the anti-hocus-pocus camp. So, am I a hypocrite? Sure, why not? As Uncle Ralph used to say, "A foolish consistency is the hobgoblin of little minds, adored by little statesmen and philosophers and divines."

I claim the right to call Ralph Waldo Emerson "Uncle Ralph" because, in our family tree, a few generations back, he was one of the cousins. Frankly, I'm thrilled he's in the family because he did some things that I greatly admire.

For one, in his early days, when he was a minister, it occurred to him that maybe the bread and wine didn't actually turn into the literal body and blood of Christ, as in the doctrine of trans-substantiation. He didn't like giving communion and mouthing words he didn't believe. So he asked his congregation if they would mind awfully much if he skipped serving communion in the church. They minded, so Uncle Ralph quit the ministry. A man of principle.

He also supported American Indian rights way back in the 1800's. He was opposed to the forced march of the Cherokees, which came to be known as the Trail of Tears, and he agitated against it, obviously unsuccessfully, but he tried. He also invited the amazing Paiute princess, Sarah Winnemucca Hopkins, to speak in his home on behalf of the rights of her people. If you don't know who she is, as soon as you've finished reading up on Sacajawea, check out her autobiography, *Life among the Piutes: Their Wrongs and Claims.* She was one fine and dedicated lady.

Before I retired, a central theme in my legal career was holding our government's feet to the fire for its wrongdoings. I'm glad to see that I came by it naturally. I salute you, Uncle Ralph.

Of course I can't claim personal pride in this famous relative's accomplishments, but I do feel an uncanny kinship. For more than a year, I logged my dreams when I awoke in the morning. I enjoy my colorful, lively dreams, but they fade rapidly, and I didn't want to lose them. I also wanted to see what I might learn about myself from them. I found out later that Uncle Ralph also used to log his dreams for the same reasons. He was exploring how his own mind worked. How many people pop out of bed first thing to log their dreams? I bet if he were alive today, he would be constantly noodling over the speed of light.

Another thing I like about him was his longevity. He was 89 when he died. I hope I got some of those genes.

But I digress. I was talking about rattling my tumor away. This was only one of the ways I participated in my own health care. There were many. In order to recover from illness, grab anything that seems to help. Soak up the kind thoughts that come with others' prayers whether or not you believe in prayer. Wallow in the beauties of nature. Swallow your stubborn independence, and accept the help that friends and family offer. Get moving with yoga, bowling, tap dancing—whatever floats your boat. Drift on a cloud of music. Laugh your guts out. Eat what you love, but love food that's fresh and real and close to the earth. Soak in a tub. Meditate. Surprise yourself with something new; go to a garden club or go to a strip club——whichever is out of character. Stir it up. Above all, let your orgasms melt your bones.

Get out of yourself with movies, art, books. Give to others what you can, when you can, but carefully. When energy wanes, don't let others steal it. Healing can be a selfish time. Forget the brave face and the endless chores. Prop up the pillows on the couch, grab a soft blankie, and put a sappy vintage movie in the DVD player.

Make a plan. I bought a season ski pass in advance, even

though I thought I might die before winter. I keep taking Italian classes for my some-day trip to Italy. In my cancer support group I'm told that making plans sends messages to the cells of my body that I expect to live. Come on cells, get with the program.

Here's what I did to enjoy my time after surgery, back when I wasn't capable of much. This is from an email I wrote to friends and family.

August 23, 2008: I need to thank all of you for the outpouring of support that helped me through my surgery and recovery. All the emails, calls, cards, visits, and oncology jokes have given my spirits a tremendous lift.

The surgery went just fine–tumor chopped out of there and shipped off to France. The recovery was a bit slow in the hospital–my digestive tract wasn't crazy about "waking up" after being severed, but once it did, I've been bouncing back rapidly. I've been home for over a week, and I take daily short walks, go up and down stairs, eat almost normally and laze around at will. I try for a short trip away from home each day. Best of all, my anemia's gone.

Thanks to Mom, stepdad Frank, sister Cathy, and niece Elizabeth, I'm getting well fed and pampered.

Next stage: I see my oncologist in early September and will find out the schedule of my treatments for the inoperable junk in my chest.

It is a lovely, late summer here in New Hampshire, with birdies chirping and bears raiding Mom and Frank's bird feeder and snakes sunning themselves on the brick floor of the greenhouse and flowers galore in Frank's gorgeous garden. Fresh berries and veggies from the local farmstands and from friends' gardens make "eating locally" a breeze. Life is good and don't let anybody tell you it ain't.

Speaking of oncology jokes. I did receive some from my friends. Such jokes are few and far between. I guess people don't think cancer's funny. Here's a sampling of what my friends dug up for me:

Doctor: "I've got very bad news–you've got cancer and Alzheimer's."

Patient: "Well, at least I don't have cancer."

Imagine this as a cartoon drawing: The oncologist is standing beside an empty bed, saying, "Good news, this time we've gotten it all!"

What do you call a person who has a compulsion to get lymphoma over and over again? A lymphomaniac.

What do you call a doctor who is always on the telephone? An on-call-ogist.

What do you call bugs with cancer? MalignANT and BEEnign.

Here are lyrics to a song that was found on the Internet:

We praise the colorectal surgeon,

Misunderstood and much maligned,

Slaving away in the heart of darkness,

Working where the sun don't shine.

Here's a joke from a relative who is a veterinarian:

A man goes to a vet's office carrying his dog. The vet examines the dog and pronounces the dog dead.

The man is upset and demands a second opinion. The vet brings in a cat, who sniffs the body, looks at the vet and meows. The vet says, "I'm sorry, but the cat agrees that your dog is dead."

The man is still unwilling to accept the news. The vet brings in a Labrador retriever. The Lab sniffs the body, looks at the vet, and barks. The vet says, "I'm sorry, but this dog agrees that your dog is dead."

The man finally accepts the diagnosis, thanks the vet and asks how much he owes. The vet answers, "$550."

"$550 to tell me my dog is dead?" exclaimed the man.

"Well," the vet replies, "I would have charged only $50 for my initial diagnosis. The additional $500 was for the cat scan and lab test."

I chuckle now when I read in my August, 2008 email, "the recovery was a bit slow in the hospital." No kidding. I was supposed to be home in five days, but stayed hospitalized for nine. After bowel surgery, your digestive system conks out and it takes time before it will process food. Mine stayed on strike. I could only swab my mouth with ice water for eight days. I was told to walk, so I pushed my pain pole around the nursing station, shuffling along in slippers and a cotton johnny. I would see trays of food for other patients, and wondered whether I would ever get to eat again.

All that time, fluid dripped into my arm. I assumed they were feeding me. At the end, I asked the doctor how many calories I had been getting and he said, "None." Zero calories for eight days. It was a potassium solution. My gut was so puffed out that I never felt hungry. Hell of a way to diet.

Surgery that extensive hurts. They gave me access to intravenous pain medication which hung from my pain pole. I could push my own button whenever I needed some. Trouble is, opiates constipate you. And we're trying to wake up the digestive tract, not put it to sleep. Thus five days of hospitalization stretched to nine.

The scar on my stomach starts above my belly button, curves around one side of it, and snakes down several more inches. I can go to Egypt without getting lost because I have a map of the

Nile on my tummy. The only good news is that I was forbidden to do sit-ups.

I don't remember how I passed all that time. I never left the ward except once on a gurney for an x-ray. I memorized every sign posted on every bulletin board as I walked 'round and 'round the nurses' station.

Visitors came and went. Mostly I enjoyed the visits, but I was vague about whom I had seen and when. People told me I was tough. People told me I was cheerful. Then my sister came to visit. She knows me better. I cried and couldn't stop. I didn't want to stop. Her presence was like a soft, warm, grandma's lap, and it was finally okay to cry. I'm looking back now into that hospital room and I see myself sitting in a big, reclining chair and I'm crying and we're saying, "This stinks." We knew that, even with all the drama from surgery, I still had that other, inoperable tumor. We knew I would probably die of it. I didn't want to leave her or Elizabeth, whom I had helped raise. We knew I had some time, but we didn't know how much. She said we still had some skiing to do. I said, yes, we did. We both cried.

Staff came and went, day and night. I liked the morning visits by the team of what I called the baby docs. Dartmouth-Hitchcock is a teaching hospital and a flock of docs who studied with my surgeon surrounded my bed each morning to check on me. The eager faces of all those darling young men were pleasant to wake up to. Girls too, but I prefer boys in my bedroom in the morning.

I developed a bond with one student from India who had followed my case before, during, and after the surgery. I gave him a little present. It was an article from a tabloid paper about a woman who puffed up and spontaneously exploded while in church. The article claimed that her flying body parts knocked her pastor out of the pulpit. Since my bowels had not moved,

I, too, was puffed up like a blowfish. I told him the article was meant as a warning if they couldn't fix me.

One day in the hospital I danced. I had a CD player, and I put on Jimi Hendrix. I closed the door to my room and cranked up the volume. I stood in my hospital johnny and swayed side to side, barely shuffling my feet, as the strong refrain from *Fire* rocked me. I know how to play that song. I used to perform it on my Fender Stratocaster, screeching feedback and all. I played air guitar while I danced, careful not to get tangled in all the tubes coming into me from my pain pole.

I was transported, not to my own performances but to the Monterrey Pops Festival in the summer of 1967, the famous Summer of Love. I was there when Jimi lit his guitar on fire. As I swayed side to side in my hospital room, I let all the light and energy and brilliance of that transformative summer pour into me. I was dancing with the colorfully clad crowds at free rock concerts in Golden Gate Park. I was sleeping in the back of a beat-up station wagon with Rusty. I was on Cannery Row in a dockside dive crashing with hippies I'd met on the street. I was clad in velvet and denim, rhinestones and paisley, dancing at the Fillmore and the Avalon.

In the hospital, I danced for my life. As I danced, poignant memories tumbled one on top of the other. I have lived hard and well. I have lived in a teepee and an Airstream trailer and a one-room cabin in the woods. I have passed a joint to Jerry Garcia. He once sang to me, "Somebody dance with the lady with the skinny legs." I always danced. I danced while Janis Joplin screamed out her soul. I danced while The Who smashed their guitars. I danced while my friend, John, sat by the entrance to the Monterrey Pops Festival passing out free LSD. This is my life, and I am celebrating it here and now, in this hospital, with Jimi cranked to the max.

Jimi is gone now. He didn't make it much past Woodstock.
Janis died too, back in the '70s. I don't know about Jimi's
overdose, but I know a guy who got heroin from the same batch
as Janis's. It was too pure and he overdosed, but he lived to
tell about it. She didn't. Jimi and Janis and Jerry injected me
with enough joy and energy to carry me through the years, but
they all died. I'm alive. I got to live a whole, rich law career
and to immerse myself in the Spanish-speaking world and play
screeching guitar, and dance, dance, dance. I've lived a long and
joyous life. I'm so glad to be here, alive, in my hospital gown,
dancing, while Jimi plays *Fire*.

On the seventh day, Connie's bowel rested. On the eighth,
it awoke. I ate some grey oatmeal. Oh, yum. On the ninth day,
I discarded my johnny and put on street clothes. I hugged
my surgeon and thanked him for saving my life. He stiffened
on being touched by a patient. To him, I was just a walking
stomach——plumbing he had repaired. To me he was a white
knight, a prince, a savior. Please, doctor, let me send gratitude
from my still-beating heart to yours. He couldn't duck my
embrace, and he finally smiled.

I walked, free of my pain pole, out of the ward. In a stretch
of hallway I hadn't yet walked, there were new and different
pictures to look at on the wall. They were the most beautiful
things I'd ever seen. I thought I was in the Hermitage Museum.
I was thrilled by all the new faces of different people. Not all of
them wore scrubs. People in street clothes. How novel.

I walked, very slowly on shaky legs, down a flight of stairs.
I saw a door to the outdoors. I went through it. The air outside
was crammed full of summer. The sweet scent of fresh mown
grass. Flowerbeds a mosaic of brilliant hues. Cloudless sky the
color of our '56 Plymouth. I no longer smelled cleaning products
mixed with plastics mixed with my own stinking bowels that

had finally let loose, turning my bathroom into an unendurable hell hole.

I stood outside the hospital looking back at the building. There was my wing. That must be my floor. Oh yes, there's my window. I recognize the flowers my brother brought me. Purple and white orchids. So delicate. There's my Teddy bear in the window. Actually it's Mom's. I gave it to her to cuddle during her mastectomy. She loaned it back to me for my bowel surgery. It was good holding Teddy to my stomach. When I walked in circles around the ward, I pushed the pain pole with one hand and clutched Teddy to my tummy with the other. He kept my stitched-together guts from jiggling painfully. At night he stayed cradled in my arms during my fitful sleeping. I would wake up disoriented, in pain, checking the hospital's wall clock in the dim light, wondering why only forty-five minutes had passed since I last checked. Then I'd clutch the softness of Teddy and doze off again.

Oh, my god. I lived an entire lifetime up there. Nine days in an endless bubble of time, not sure I would ever leave. But I made it out. I'm on the outside now, looking back in.

◇◇◇◇◇

Chapter Nine

While I was driving east from Devils Tower, the weather turned cold and windy, with scattered rain. The sky was wide open, with miles to the horizon. Clouds clustered into gloomy, dark masses, too thick to hold the mist airborne. It streaked to the ground in grey swaths. In every direction, scattered veils of grey dropped from the sky while glowing sun punched through in patches; the whole sky a panoramic dance of light and shadow.

I entered the Black Hills National Forest. In the famous Wild West town of Deadwood, South Dakota, I found a KOA campground. I planned to pitch my tent there, but their basic log cabins caught my eye. Very basic. The bathrooms were in a distant building. The cabins had little more than a bare bed and a light bulb. The big draw? A heater. Oh yeah. I was happy to pay the extra fee for a cabin on this frigid night. I'll also pause here to offer a prayer of thanks to the inventor of the insulating fabric, Polarfleece.

The town of Deadwood has been immortalized in so many westerns with Wild Bill Hickok, Doc Holliday, and Calamity Jane that I doubt anybody can sort fiction from history anymore. In 1959, Deadwood was a fun spot for kids. Every cutesy, western gimmick was easily marketed to our unsophisticated tastes. It was a simpler era. We could pretend to pan for gold and we could hear honky tonk piano music coming out of fake bars that had swinging wooden doors. A cartoon caricature of the Wild West.

Deadwood has changed. By 1990 it was a dying town. The buildings in Deadwood are great examples of massive stone, frontier architecture, but the buildings were crumbling. Since the entire town is a historic district, the local citizenry convinced the state legislature that part of their legitimate history was, of course, gambling. So they've converted most of the buildings to casinos. No more kids in red felt cowboy hats.

The gambling revenue exceeded all expectations, and the buildings in the town are all spruced up now. The casinos are as nice inside as casinos get. Plenty of room and not too smoky. There are table games, and all kinds of slot machines, including the increasingly popular penny slots, where you can sometimes stretch twenty or thirty dollars into an evening's entertainment if you keep your bets low enough. You'll never win much, but you won't have to pawn your wedding ring.

I enjoyed plinking around on the penny slots where I won some and lost some, and ended up contributing my fair share to the town coffers. You may well ask, "What's fun about penny slots?" I'll tell you. They are silly children's video games for grownups–a complete waste of time and money. That's precisely their appeal. You can feel decadent for an hour or two without risking your child's college tuition. It's a tame taste of sin, but it is gambling, and gambling is addictive, so watch out.

I got served free diet colas while playing, and I ate a discounted buffet dinner. I was glad to be indoors, out of the cold, but wondered, where are all the dancing girls and the shootouts in the street? It's the Tame, Tame West.

In the morning I took the road from Deadwood to the Mt. Rushmore National Memorial. It went through a high, forested area of rolling hills, which is a scenic route on the AAA map, but which is marred by tacky tourist attractions and infested with bilious billboards. There's even a carnival with a perpetually spinning Ferris wheel enticing children to whine and fuss until Daddy stops the car.

Worse yet is the town of Keystone near Mt. Rushmore. Keystone is a hideous concoction brewed of avarice and tastelessness into an eye-jarring jumble of Wild West tourist traps. It was the off-season, so, thankfully, I didn't get stuck in traffic there, where I would have been forced to look at the place.

At Mt. Rushmore, my senior pass was no advantage, because they allow a private concession to soak everybody for ten bucks to park in an urban-looking, multi-level parking garage. A far cry from the fifties when you just parked near the cafeteria and gift shop. And an even farther cry from when my mother visited in the thirties. Her photos show the face of George Washington mostly finished. And the other faces? Not even begun. Now in 2009, there is a triumphant arched entryway sporting the flags of all fifty states, a large cafeteria, a massive gift shop, a museum, a visitors center, and the sculptor's workshop. Oh, and if you have a spare minute to look up, you might see some faces carved on a mountain.

I was prepared to be unimpressed with this star-spangled icon of unabashed patriotism, but I'll admit right now, the four smooth, solemn faces emerging from the jagged rocks are such a feat of massive portraiture that I was amazed at the workmanship. The phenomenal feat of putting these things up there temporarily trumped my cynicism.

Why cynicism? Think about it. Most monumental sculptures that last through the ages are of gods, or are tributes to powerful kings that ruled for a lifetime. Think of the Sphinx, or of the monumental Buddhas that stood for centuries in a cliff in Afghanistan until the Taliban blew the beautiful sculptures to kingdom come. Assholes. But the point is, when folks go to all the trouble of carving images that could last for thousands of years, as these Mt. Rushmore faces are expected to do, people preserve what they believe to be universally important figures.

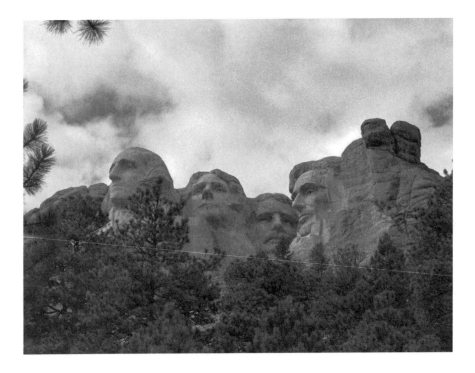

So, who do we get? Four government bureaucrats who, for no more than eight years apiece, presided over the executive branch of our tri-pillared government, then retired to play golf (except for the one who got assassinated first). It's not that surprising that many visitors know little about the four chosen presidents. Pop quiz: name the four presidents on Mt. Rushmore. Give up? You've got lots of company. As I was examining the visages, one man asked me, "Who is the one with the mustache?" He was referring to Teddy Roosevelt, famous for his support of national parks. The other three are Washington, Jefferson and Lincoln, each of whom presided during major turning points in U.S. history. We can endure gazing at their faces only because they've been dead a long time. Can you imagine looking up there at Gerald Ford or Jimmy Carter? Get real.

The idea of sticking presidents' heads on a mountainside came from one local guy with the unabashed motive of attracting tourism to the Black Hills. Boy, did he succeed. But the monument does capture something of the American spirit. It is decidedly secular and civic, reminding us of the important principles of freedom and democracy (Washington and Jefferson), equality (Lincoln), and love for our purple mountains' majesty (Roosevelt), even if it is the height of white male hubris to carve up the whole purple mountain.

Before walking the circular trail that leads close to the faces, I ate lunch in the cafeteria, which has oversized, round tables, so you are invited to sit with strangers. I liked this idea. I chose a table with a group of retired, black tourists who had traveled together on a bus from Tennessee. They asked me if I had seen the Smoky Mountains, and I related a tale of our car breaking down in a remote part of the Smokies, and how we finally made it to an isolated farmhouse where the owner happened to be a car mechanic. He was wonderfully helpful, but we could hardly understand each other, our accents were so different. One black woman said, in her lovely, lilting drawl, "A real hillbilly, huh?" I wasn't going to be so politically incorrect as to say it, but she nailed it.

I enjoyed sitting in the midst of their humorous chit-chat filled with teasing banter. It was clear they enjoyed each other's company on their tour, except for one complaining biddy who could have formed the prototype for the self-righteous sister-in-law on the old sitcom, Sanford and Son. I imagined this pinch-faced woman in an oversized hat at her church, harping on about everyone's faults. There's a spoilsport in every crowd.

I walked the circular trail that brings you right under the big cheeses' noses. The angles keep changing as you get closer, and the scale of these huge faces gets more impressive. By the time you are practically beneath them, you could look up and see their boogers, if the carvings were truly realistic.

Just off the footpath were two, long-haired, gleaming-white mountain goats. They calmly posed for photos. One resolute photographer kept creeping closer until he was only five or six feet from one of the mountain goats, in violation of the rule about staying distant from wildlife. A passing tourist said to me, "I bet that goat would enjoy seeing his pal butt that guy." I said, "*I'd* enjoy seeing that."

There was a life-sized replica of an Indian village. The day-to-day artifacts were on display including a teepee with a fire pit in the center. It looked cozy and familiar. In the summer of 1969, right after my college graduation, I moved with Good Dog North into a teepee in the woods in Estacada, Oregon, where I lived for the summer.

We had a small, hippy-style community there. There were a couple of rented farmhouses, and at the end of a long trail into the woods, beside a gurgling stream, was a vacant teepee where Bob and Barbara let me stay. The teepee was big enough to sleep crowds of people. It hosted one large, LSD-charged gathering of the half-clad and the unclad that summer. That's what things were like back then. Loosey goosey, for sure.

I learned to appreciate the perfect design of a teepee. There's a smoke hole at the peak where the wooden tent poles cross. By leaving the opening flap slightly ajar, you get cross-ventilation, and it's safe from carbon-monoxide poisoning when a fire is burning in the central fire pit. Starting from halfway up the walls, a separate flap of canvas hangs down inside, creating a layer of air between the outer wall and the inner lining. This insulates the teepee, and, with a good fire, you stay warm in the coldest weather. Rain runs down ridges in the poles and then runs off at the edges. The inside stays dry. Ours was made of canvas, but the originals were made from animal hides. When the plains Indians needed to move, they would pack up the teepees, and their horses would drag the poles along, so they were portable out in the plains. In the woods, not so much. The Indians in the wooded areas of Oregon built large, rectangular longhouses.

I admired the teepee, and told the ranger that I used to live in one. No reaction. Except mine was much bigger, I bragged. The young ranger looked at me like, "Yeah, right." I thought, "Honest, ranger. I did live in a great big teepee. It was terrific. You should try it sometime."

After leaving Mt. Rushmore, I rapidly passed through Rapid City, South Dakota and noticed some seedy casinos there, not as elegant as Deadwood's. One advertised that they cash paychecks. I was stunned. I'm no prude, but even I can see the evil in that. There oughta be a law. Anybody so gripped with a vicious gambling addiction that he'd rush in to have his paycheck cashed in a casino, where he'll promptly lose junior's milk money, should not be taken advantage of like that.

Next stop was Wall, South Dakota, home of the famous Wall Drug. The store is so famous, it has its own Wikipedia entry. Starting from hundreds of miles away, billboards proclaim the myriad wonders of Wall Drug. "See the animated, smoke-puffing dinosaur!" "See thousands of Wild West photos!" Here's the one that grabbed me: "Five-cent coffee and homemade doughnuts." Guess I'll be stopping at Wall Drug.

Although it consists of a sprawling series of shops that peddle western dust-catchers made in China, the doughnuts alone are worth the stop. They have thin, crispy crusts that crunch ever so slightly when you bite, while the insides are fluffy and cake-like. These doughnuts lack the cloying greasiness of that brand whose name hints that you should dunk them in your coffee.

Along with a five-cent cup of good coffee, all I can say is, I'm glad I lived long enough to bite this food.

What made me linger for a good part of the afternoon, and even to return in the morning for a second look (and a second doughnut), was the astonishing display of close to 2,000 historical photographs. They appear everywhere throughout the store. The back room is crammed frame to frame on a long wall that runs for the better part of a city block. If a picture is worth a thousand words, a good, long look at this collection will substitute for a library full of books on western history. You can see the real Annie Oakley, Calamity Jane, and Buffalo Bill looking right at you.

One of the photographers who captured many of these priceless images was a man named John Anderson. He was born in Sweden in 1869 and began taking photographs for the U.S. Army in 1885. He became the owner of a trading post on the Rosebud Reservation in 1893, and for forty-two years he lived among and photographed the Broulé Sioux, capturing images of their everyday life as well as their stunning regalia. A book of his photos, now out of print, but available used through Amazon.com is by Henry Hamilton, called *The Sioux of the Rosebud: A History in Pictures*.

These images show Indians at home in their camps, with their horses, teepees, and dogs. It shows them hunting and cooking. The photos are hanging on the wall in uneasy juxtaposition with photos of white homesteaders, the famous sodbusters who took advantage of the government's land giveaway, intended to spur settlement, only to discover that the limited acreage on parched land was too little for survival. Many packed up and headed to pastures that were literally greener in Oregon and California. The sodbusters stand beside their partially underground, sod homes looking at the camera lenses with lean and solemn faces, holding the hands of their scrawny, barefoot children dressed in rags. Later in history, they are replaced by well-heeled settlers–the women dressed in fur coats and muffs–the horses well-fed and pulling nicely-built carriages.

The facial structure of the plains Indians fascinates me. These photos show the craggy faces of famous chiefs with their classic, eagle feather headdresses, and also lesser known braves. These faces–with long, beaked noses, as regal as any Roman emperor's, and with high, pronounced cheekbones, piercingly clear eyes, and golden skin–what roots do these folk spring from?

Most Indian mythology has them springing from whatever ground they inhabit now. I suppose some Indians still believe this, but if I were an Indian, I'd want to know the history of the migrations of my ancestors. Before some of the southern tribes settled down to grow corn, they were all nomadic hunter-gatherers, and most engaged in warfare and slavery, so, almost certainly there would have been plenty of wandering as they competed for resources.

I'm also not that impressed with the archeologists and anthropologists on this point. They theorize that the indigenous people of America *all* came from a band or bands of Asians who strolled across a then-existing northern land bridge into Alaska and then southward. But I wonder whether ten or twelve thousand years is long enough to account for the widely different physiognomies we see in the Americas. There are lanky, plains Indians with their Roman noses and long-straight hair, there are short, round-faced Indians with barrel-shaped torsos, there are lean-faced Indians with the flat foreheads of their Aztec ancestors, there are diminutive Indians with kinky hair in the rain forests of South America. The long-lost Olmecs in Mexico carved faces with broad, African-type noses and thick lips. Indigenous eyes can be round, or can have tucked flaps, Chinese style. There are a wide range of skin colors. So my question has always been, since indigenous Americans don't look closely related, might they have different genetic roots? If that's the case, how and when did their ancestors get here?

I'm thinking boats. Maybe simple basket boats. As soon as you figure out how to weave a basket, you might notice that it floats. If you seal it up with something sticky like pitch, it doesn't leak. The Vietnamese still use lovely, round basket boats that must be of ancient origin. Say you've got enough gourds full of water and you've got your dried meat, and your boat drifts off course. Or else you committed a crime, so your tribe pushes you and your little basket boat out to sea, warning you there's a spear with your name on it if you return. You drift off, never knowing on what shore you'll wash up. People might have drifted here from just about anyplace that has a seashore. Sure, most would have drowned, but it only takes a couple of breeders who make it, and the rest is pre-history.

This is all, of course, just another of my wild, unsubstantiated theories. There are genetic studies going on now to map early human migration patterns. I hope they're done before I die. Just one more enticement to keep living.

I may be wrong, but not so wrong as those who add up all the Biblical "begats" since Adam and Eve to reach the conclusion that the earth is only 6,000 years old. It's a wonderful thing that creation myths told around ancient campfires have been preserved for millennia. We should treasure those stories, but believing their literal truth in light of easy-to-access scientific information is a bad case of willful ignorance.

Returning to the photos in the back room at Wall Drug, one chilling photo shows a grainy image of a soldier standing over snow-covered corpses of Lakota Sioux Indians at the famous Wounded Knee Massacre, or Battle of Wounded Knee, depending on who's telling the story. After enough broken treaties, and after the gold-rushing whites pushed the Indians out of their sacred Black Hills, a group of Ghost Dancers formed the belief that they could dance the whites off their lands. In 1890, the U.S. government proved they couldn't by slaughtering three hundred Sioux men, women, and children at Wounded Knee. Government casualties? Something like twenty-five or twenty-six, many of whom were probably killed in the U.S. crossfire.

I've always been disturbed by photographs of real people who are really dead. I remember watching World War II documentaries on television during the 1950's in which airplanes were shot out of the sky, and I, a child in grade school, was well aware that they held real humans who were dying before our eyes. I couldn't understand how my family could calmly watch these scenes while the announcer droned on about victory over the enemy. I still can't.

The soldier in the Wounded Knee photo is too grainy for us to read his expression. Is this a proud trophy photo? Is he at all saddened by the carnage? We'll never know.

Back in a far corner, near the Wall Drug bathrooms, there's a series of five photos depicting more death. It is a rare sequence of photos of a public hanging. They show the hanging of Earnest Loveswar in Sturgis, South Dakota, on September 19, 1902, for the murders of George Puck and Henry Ostrander. This was the last public hanging in Meade County.

Loveswar was an Indian, and Puck and Ostrander were white homesteaders. Makes me want to re-open his case to look for any prejudice, not that an Indian can't kill white guys, but I'd bet my law degree that if there were mitigating circumstances, the jurors never heard them.

Earnest Loveswar is all dressed up for his hanging in a nice suit and tie. In photo number one, the presiding dignitaries are walking him up the stairs of the wooden scaffolding. In numbers two and three, they appear to be posing for the photos. If I had to guess, I'd say it's got to be the Sheriff, the mayor, and maybe a state legislator up there taking advantage of the photo-op. Young Mr. Loveswar displays the same facial expression they do; serious, but not terrified. It's as if he knows his role. *I'm the guy they're hanging, so I must act dignified up here.*

In photo number four, they bind his arms and legs. He looks down at what they are doing with apparent calm, as if his only thought is to make certain they get it right.

In photo number five, you see the backs of the heads of the men in the crowd. Just past them is a silhouetted human shape hanging by the neck underneath the scaffolding. Goodbye, Earnest Loveswar.

Although we no longer have public hangings in the United States, we still administer the death penalty. We are the last of the so-called developed nations to do so. Mexico, for example, thinks we're barbaric. They got rid of their death penalty ages ago. That's all I'll say about that. Don't get me started. This book isn't long enough for my opinion about government-sponsored murder.

Death. First you're here, and then you're not. It's inconceivable, incomprehensible, an eternal puzzle how that can be. Even birds are stunned by the mystery of death. I still mourn a bird that I hit with my car in 1984. That's twenty-five years ago. I heard something hit the windshield and I saw a dark flash of movement out of the corner of my eye. I slowed to a stop and looked back. There was a dead bird in the street. Its mate flew to it and stood beside it. It just stayed there, looking at its sweetheart, dead in the street. *Why can't my love fly anymore? Get up, darling. Let's fly.* My heart still aches for both of them.

Last year, I thought I would die soon. I thought I would be here, and then I would not be here. I thought my friends and family would be confused. Puzzled. Where did she go? She came from a whole line of life, starting from the beginning of life itself, uninterrupted. My parents came from their parents who came from their parents. I picture a little piece of continuous life inside each ancestor; a string of life that ties me to the first cell that ever divided. Life, uninterrupted for billions of years. In my DNA I literally carry the encyclopedia of life from the very start. My brain remembers only this life, but my cells know my history starting from the ancient past. But, one day, my continuous lifeline will be gone in a moment. Ended. What a weird way to run a world.

I'd be shocked to wake up after death in some stranger's version of heaven. In the West, we usually say we have one soul, and it goes to whatever place our various religions have dreamed up. The old Norse heaven, Valhalla, was interesting. After death, the warriors fought all day, and if they were lucky, they got killed so they could rise up and go to a banquet and feast all night and go do battle again the next day. For eternity. I don't get how, if you're already dead, you can get killed repeatedly in heaven, or why you would want to, but that's their story.

I'm not sure what advantage the women got in Valhalla, but they apparently wanted to go there if their husbands or masters were killed. I once read a Roman's eyewitness account of a Norse slave girl who supposedly volunteered to be sacrificed after her master died. So they gave her a feast, got her all doped up, and when she was too goofy to protest, they hung her by the neck and stabbed her in the chest. I'm glad to live in an era when human sacrifice has gone out of style.

Modern religious conceptions of the afterlife are also

strange—attentive virgins for the Muslim men, but what exactly do the women get? Beats me.

In some eastern religions a person has two or more souls. One goes to heaven and the other hangs around on earth as a ghost and usually wreaks havoc. Ancestor worship is as much about placating the restless souls as it is about revering them.

Christianity turns out to have several versions of heaven depending on the passage of scripture you're reading, but you're pretty sure to run into Jesus, a heavenly host of angels, and God the Father. It is widely believed that music there will sound like the Mormon Tabernacle Choir singing Handel's *Messiah*. And if you're Mormon, you add all your relatives into the mix. Mormon heaven is heavily populated.

It's all puzzling to me. I see Alzheimer's patients lose themselves even before they die, so I wonder why human egos universally insist that our private personalities will transcend death after all the wiring that maintains our quirks and idiosyncrasies has shut down. Many people find comfort in an afterlife where they remain in some conscious form. Frankly, that terrifies me. I'd prefer eternal rest. Lights out. It strikes me as a better deal. I've always been a busy person, and I'd rather not keep doing stuff after I die. I crave a long nap. But if there's a massive and eternal Q consciousness out there, like on Star Trek, and if I must return to the Q collective after death, I hope to meet the virile captain of the Enterprise, Jean-Luc Picard. That would make heaven bearable.

I don't fear the part of death that happens after I die. I believe I won't be aware of anything at all. There's a time every night, during deep sleep, when we don't dream. Scientists have put electrodes on peoples' heads to determine this. Our autonomic nervous system keeps the factory humming—heart keeps beating, lungs keep breathing—but mentally there's nobody home. I don't mind going there every night. Total ego loss. Complete lack of awareness. It happens every single night, and doesn't hurt a bit. I suspect death will be like that.

Similarly, although there are proponents of the theory that we have lived past lives, if I did so, I don't remember them. As far as I'm concerned, there were billions of years before my birth when I was not invited to the party. I imagine death as another long, non-party time.

But I do have a dread, sometimes a terror, of dying. Our bodies are built to go to any extreme to stay alive. If my body is fighting to live, and something is fighting to kill me, that battlefield can be a living hell. I've already tasted a bit of it. I don't want that agony, and if I must have it, I hope it's mercifully short. I might live an entire life filled mostly with joy and light and laughter only to suffer horribly in the end. That's my biggest fear.

I have ways to calm my own fears. Clutching Teddy in the long, restless nights after surgery helped a bit. Rattling my African rattle over my tumor helped calm me. I know how to meditate, and I go there sometimes. Breathe deeply. Let all thoughts pass through the mind without latching onto them. Watch the calm glow in the center of my forehead. I have used guided meditation that comes on CD's. I let the recorded voice talk me into envisioning a quiet spot in nature where all is peaceful and lovely. These things work.

That is, they work except for the times when I've been so mentally out of it that I can't begin to seek comfort in any of them. Maybe there are accomplished yogis who can meditate their way past some of the worst tricks our sick bodies can play on us, but I'm not one of them. I remember when I was in the hospital getting nasty interleukin-2 treatments. On television, the hospital's programming showed a station with pictures of nature at her most lovely while a soundtrack played soft music. This was the hospital's way of giving us a chance at calming ourselves during trying times. I would put on that channel, but the interleukin made me agitated and fearful. It was so overwhelming that I was only aware of a bright light above my bed with flashing colors on it. I vaguely remember sounds, and knew it was music, but it felt so far away it couldn't touch me. You can't use positive imaging techniques when your own brain can't identify them. That's why I fear, not death, but dying. I hate being flung into anguish with no way to stop the horror.

Chapter Ten

It's hard to believe that only one year before my cross-country camping trip I was in Dartmouth-Hitchcock hospital getting pumped full of interleukin-2. I had to wait six weeks after my summertime surgery to get strong enough for my next medical clobbering, so it was well into September of 2008 before I checked back in for the first of two rounds of IL-2.

During the six weeks between the surgery and the first IL-2 treatment, I spent a curiously sweet time. My fear of death was constant, but it was background noise. Impending death seemed inevitable, but there was summer to enjoy. And my life as an invalid had a strangely relaxing quality. Nobody expected me to do anything, so I did nothing. When I wanted a popsicle, I piped up from my permanent station on the couch, "Can somebody get me a popsicle?" Somebody always did. You can't get away with that crap when you feel well.

Back in the sixties, when I was living off of not much more than air and brown rice, I noticed that only the very rich and the very poor have much leisure time to enjoy. Now I add the infirm to that list. It's not exactly enjoyment when accompanied by pain, but my summertime walks were special. A hike on a mountain trail is invigorating, but, under normal conditions, I tend to rush past the lovely details of all the growth in the forest. After surgery, my walks were more like the ones in my childhood when I used to walk ever so slowly with my grandmother. I went at her slow pace because my legs were so short they couldn't cover much ground no matter how fast I pumped them. The attractions during those childhood walks were stones and berries and pine cones—all the little things that a small hand could grasp for closer examination.

During my summer walks after the operation, I would stop to pick a dandelion and watch with fascination as its white fluff dislodged from the stem and drifted like Tinkerbell on a warm breeze. I would go down to the frog pond and watch patiently for bubbles. Then I'd notice two moist eyes poking above the surface of the water. Ribbit. I would go to the greenhouse and watch snakes warming their bellies on the hot floor and marvel at the intact shells of skin from which they'd managed to wriggle. The lilies in my stepfather's garden emitted sweet, concentrated perfume. Walking with cautious baby steps forced me to linger long enough to fill my lungs with their precious scent. Like a four-year-old, I discovered a world of wonder right outside our door.

A friend had planted a garden. When I needed an outing, he brought me to where his tomatoes had gobbled up enough summer sunshine that they burst with orange-red juice, sweeter than store-bought tomatoes. His runaway pumpkins made me laugh. Didn't they know he'd fenced the garden? What were pumpkins doing all over the dirt road? He picked up logs off his woodpile and showed me where snakes were hiding. The wood absorbed heat from the sun, and the spaces between the logs made safe havens. Those were some happy, warm snakes.

Before going back into the hospital, I made it to a few of Colleen's exercise classes in the Town Hall, but I modified everything. With my innards barely intact, I was forbidden to do sit-ups. Instead of jogging in place with the others, I did the granny shuffle at the rear of the class. I stretched carefully. The scar was healing well, but I took no chances with any sudden movements. I sat in a chair for the hand-weight exercises, but I didn't lift any weights. I simply moved my arms as if I were holding weights. People said I was tough, but that wasn't it. I was whispering to my body, gently coaxing it back to health. *Okay, body, remember these movements? Let's get with the program. I know you can't do everything, but do what you can. Something is better than nothing.*

I don't fantasize that I can cure my own cancer by staying fit, but if exercise helps my immune system at all, that's good. And the healthier my body is going into treatment, the better off I'll be during recovery. That was my thinking.

I also went to exercise classes because it was good to see my friends again. One of them, Ann, is also a melanoma patient of Dr. Ernstoff's. She has Stage III melanoma, and he treated her, successfully so far, with interferon which is a type of immunotherapy designed to boost the immune system. It has a ton of side effects including extreme fatigue, but Ann refused to succumb to exhaustion. She walks several miles a day from her home to the town store, and she exercises three times a week in Colleen's class. She even kept up her volunteer work during her treatments. When I had to sit down to exercise, Ann was my guiding light. She's in her retirement years, and her level of fitness is great for that reason alone. But here she is, after being clobbered with interferon, bouncing up and down on her bird legs like a youngster. Colleen plays, "Oowee, oowee baby, won't you come and take me on a sea cruise," and Ann steps lively to the music. You go, girl! You give me hope.

I dubbed the two of us the Melanoma Mamas. I said we should form a rock band with that name. Now, whenever I meet other women being treated for melanoma, I invite them to join the Melanoma Mamas. We haven't yet gotten together for a band rehearsal, since we're scattered all over the globe. I've neglected to determine if any of the others play an instrument. I figure that's no problem, because they can always play kazoo or tambourine. If you're a woman and you've got melanoma, you're in. You can rock out with the Melanoma Mamas.

It was good to get out of the house to exercise class because, in that summer of 2008, the world had shrunk to the size of my hospital ward. Then it expanded to the size of my mother's house and yard. By fall, I could get out for short trips, and I noticed that there was a town full of kind people who cared about how I was doing. That's about all the progress I made before getting slammed again by the doctors.

As I mentioned before, my melanoma oncologist, Dr. Ernstoff, told me that I didn't qualify for the clinical trial where some French hotshots would have made a vaccine from my abdominal tumor. The tumor had been attached to my small intestine. It might have gotten contaminated with feces, so it couldn't be used.

Then I got all pumped about participating in a different clinical trial, but my numbers on a preliminary blood test weren't right, so I flunked out.

I was feeling gun-shy from all the mediocre medical care that I'd received during my long bout with anemia. I wanted this doctor to snap to attention. Senator Ted Kennedy had been in the news with his then recently-diagnosed brain tumor, and I had been impressed with how quickly they had run all the tests and diagnosed his condition. A sharp contrast to my own delayed diagnosis. The urgency of my condition had become clear to me, and I refused to be handled as a run-of-the-mill case anymore. I asked Dr. Ernstoff what treatment he would recommend if I were Ted Kennedy. I asked what he would do if I were his own wife. It's not that he wasn't attentive to my case. I sensed plenty of caring. But I insisted he treat me as his star patient, at least until his next star patient walked in.

I reminded Dr. Ernstoff that the inoperable tumor in my chest had been discovered in July, and it was now well into

September. I asked about standard treatments as opposed to wasting time trying to qualify for clinical trials.

That's when Dr. Ernstoff gave it to me straight. He said that interleukin-2 was an option. He said that it wouldn't kill me, but I'd wish I were dead. That's right. Those were my doctor's own words. And that turned out to be the sugar-coated version.

He told me that the chance of long-term remission after treatment was only eight percent. That means only eight of one hundred IL-2 patients regain years of life expectancy. Only twenty percent get some kind of benefit, such as slowing the tumor's growth. The rest get no benefit. We sign up for the harshest treatment possible, and most of us die within a year or so. Why do we do it? If we're going to die within a year anyway, why not shoot for the eight percent? As Bob Dylan said, "When you ain't got nothin', you got nothin' to lose."

For those who protest that doctors shouldn't poison you to cure you, and that natural remedies are kinder to the system, listen up. Interleukin-2 is a natural remedy. It is a protein we produce in our own bodies when our immune systems need a boost. It is part of our body's natural system for fighting disease. Sounds good, but just because something is natural doesn't mean it's gentle. Stand back. Here comes the IL-2. POW!

The chemistry of how it works, when it does manage to work, is far beyond me, but the general idea is that interleukin-2 massively boosts the immune system. Cancer cells hide from the immune system by pretending to be normal, healthy cells instead of ugly stuff. The immune system must first, recognize the enemy and, second, destroy it. With a massively boosted immune system, there's sufficient firepower to destroy the cancer if the immune system can find it. But it doesn't always spot the cancer, so IL-2 doesn't always work.

Since interleukin-2 offers at least a slim chance of long-term survival, I opted for it. I like life. I'll take a second helping, please. Sign me up, Doc.

Not so fast. Here's the catch. I am told I must first qualify. There are tests I must pass. My heart sank. Where have I heard this before?

Okay, let's run the tests. First, my heart. It's beating fine. Good old ticker. Now, my lungs. Up and running also.

What's this testing about? Interleukin-2 is so harsh on the system, you have to be healthy before they'll treat you with it. Excuse me, Doc? Didn't you just tell me I'm dying of cancer, and now you tell me you can't treat it unless I'm healthy? Precisely. So now I'm patting myself on the back for doing all those exercises. I passed the stress tests, and I'm in.

Administering interleukin-2 is an art form in which only a few hospitals specialize. When they first started fooling with the stuff, they killed some patients with the treatment itself. That's why they inject it while the patient is hospitalized. The specially trained medical staff constantly monitors the myriad side affects to counteract them as soon as they surface. At the first sign of major trouble, they can rush you to the intensive care unit. No kidding. It's been years since they've killed a patient. But more on these side effects later. I could write a book. Oh yeah, I am writing a book.

Here's what I remember packing for the first of my six-day hospital stays to receive IL-2 treatments. Teddy, of course. A CD player and miscellaneous music. Several CD's of guided imagery specifically for cancer patients. Sudoku puzzle books. Some books that I never read because I soon lost the necessary attention span. My African rattle that I shook over my chest to calm myself and to visualize vibrating the tumor loose. Face make-up and barrettes for my hair. Girls will be girls.

I had asked Dr. Ernstoff whether I could have visitors. He

told me that I may or may not feel like having them, but that I was permitted to have visitors twenty-four hours a day.

I said, "You mean my twenty-five-year-old Mexican pool boy can stay all night?"

He said, "I'll write it in the order."

So that's how I landed in the hospital exactly one year before my cross-country camping trip. Now, one year later, with my expiration date miraculously extended, I'm in the campground in Wall, South Dakota. The campground is mostly for R.V.'s, meaning the owners spend less attention to designing charming, rustic campsites than they do to lining up vehicles side by side with hookups for the required conveniences; water, electricity, and sewage disposal. The owners count on the campers staying inside, not noticing the dreary layout. Okay, there's a view of a grain elevator right next to the campground. That's the scenery. And there's the luxury of a pavilion beside my tent with a lightbulb, so I can see to write in my journal.

The following day's lavish scenery made up for it. I toured South Dakota's Badlands National Park. I found it stunningly gorgeous, but an appreciation of a landscape so unfriendly to human habitation is not universal. I had asked one of the locals in Wall how long it takes to tour the park. He said, "About thirty seconds." I blinked and looked puzzled. He said, "You drive to the entrance, look in, and turn around and come back." Ranchers apparently have zero use for such a parched place. Why do you think they call it badlands?

I spent more than thirty seconds in the park. Although you could drive through it in about an hour, I spent the better part of a day getting lost in reveries about tenuous life clinging to impossible cliffsides, about millions of years worth of exposed geology, and about how comical prairie dogs sound when they squeal. I had used my parks pass to get in free, so I made sure to get my money's worth.

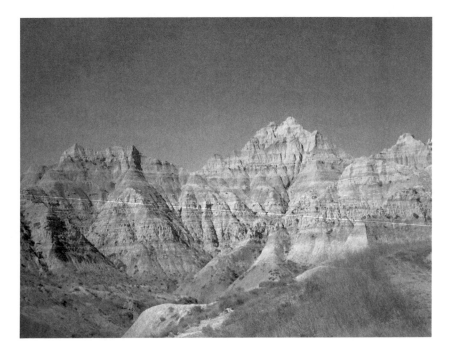

With its spiky pinnacles of striped stone, the Badlands' landscape is another American icon. It graces calendar pages and address labels and screen savers with photos that show it glowing pink at sunrise or orange at sunset. It's almost a cliché. That is, until you get there, and wowie, zowie.

The badlands are not old in geological terms. It only took about half a million years for flat plains to become eroded into this maze of phantasmagorical hills. Because the area used to be plains, some of the flat plateaus can still support enough grassland that the ranchers used to hay them, before the area became a national park. But there's no good access to those plateaus, sitting as they do on isolated hilltops, so the ranchers used to dismantle their haying machines and haul the parts up with ropes. After they had re-assembled them and finished their haying, they would attach the bales of hay to cables and let the hay slide down the cables into the canyons below. I did not learn whether any intrepid rancher ever rode down on top of the hay bales, like a primitive zip line.

On first glance, the whole area looks barren. Not much can thrive in such dry, windswept conditions, nor make it through the bitter cold winters. But a closer look reveals a variety of hardy vegetation that has learned to grow in crevices in the rocks, in shaded spots that are not scorched by sunlight, or in valleys where a bit of soil has accumulated. Desert plants are scraggly or thorny, in keeping with their need to preserve water, which would be lost through the surface of wide, green leaves. At the base of the hills where the land flattens out, even in the midst of what looks like thick grassland, you'll find nasty cactus hiding.

My family discovered this in 1959, so I went looking for the cactus this time. Back then, we had arrived late in the evening to make camp in the Badlands. It was getting dark. The grass looked benign. I remember pitching our canvas tent in one of these meadows and getting ambushed by cactus that pierced and poked right through the bottom of the tent. I recall looking at the fading light on the dry hillsides, and instead of seeing their rugged beauty, I saw unfriendly, dead rocks. I thought, "I hate this place." I could be hanging around the town pool with my pals, doing back dives off the diving board, or getting teased by one or another of the hunky Martelli cousins, or trading photos with my girlfriends to put in our miniature photo albums that we carry in our leather shoulderbags——black-and-white photos of us hugging each other in photo booths, while sticking our tongues out at the camera. But no. My family has to work on togetherness, so they squash us kids into a hot car all day for days on end, and we land up in this godforsaken desert full of hidden cactus, and now they're making us sleep on top of it. Boo hoo! I want to go home.

Isn't that just like a kid? The parents go out of their way to help us create treasured memories, and my biggest memory is getting homesick in the Badlands. But hey–it still happens. At some point during each of my marathon camping trips I've always had a Badlands moment. "This place sucks. I want to go home. What am I doing here?" Remember that part about the overpriced motel outside Yellowstone when I was dragging butt? That was this trip's Badlands moment. The only difference is that now I know I'll snap out of it. When you're twelve, it's the end of the world.

As I said, the Badlands aren't as barren as they appear. There are plenty of bugs and birds and reptiles. Even animals as large as buffalo can find enough to eat. I saw some buffalo and some of the lovely, brown and white pronghorn antelope, and a gazillion prairie dogs.

Prairie dogs burrow and then they pop up out of holes in the center of raised mounds. Then they start squealing. I stepped to the edge of a prairie dog town where dozens of them were gathered. They all started popping out of their holes and squealing at once, so no individual squeal carried much weight. In their frustration at being ignored, they hopped straight up in the air and screeched even louder. They jumped so high, I could see air beneath their feet. As they popped up and down having little prairie dog tantrums, they had me laughing out loud, (or LOL, as I wrote in my journal, evidently under the influence of my text-messaging teenage niece).

Prairie dogs are no laughing matter to the locals. I commented to a woman who worked in a mini-mart that I enjoyed seeing all the prairie dogs. She said, "We hate prairie dogs. They kill horses."

I remained speechless while I tried to figure out what she could possibly mean. I pictured a whole gang of vicious prairie dogs mobbing an unsuspecting horse and taking him down.

She saw my puzzled look and said, "The horse steps in a prairie dog hole and breaks its leg, and we have to shoot him."

I'm thinking, it's not the *prairie dog*, but the *person* who killed the horse, if you apply the *Palsgraf v. Long Island Railroad Co.* proximate cause analysis to this case. Sorry. I relapsed into legalese. But lawyers would find this funny if they had a sense of humor.

I stopped for views, and for short walks. A desert is just backdrop scenery until I walk about in it. Then the details of plants and insects and lizards begin to emerge. I watched with envy as two young backpackers headed off on a trail wearing their hiking boots, ready for a wilderness adventure. I still lacked the energy for wandering far from the road, but even a short stroll opens up new and wonderful worlds.

I walked around in a picnic area at the base of one of the cliffs, where I could examine the different plants that grow on these dry, crumbling rocks. I saw lizards scamper from where they'd been sunning themselves. The plains that stretched out at the foot of the rocks had been scorched by a wildfire. All that was left, besides some charred, blackened grass were— you guessed it—those stumpy little cacti that hide in the grass. Crowds of them everywhere, even after the fire. Those suckers are tougher than a boiled owl.

I took a civilized walk on a boardwalk built over the land. What drew me were the displays of fossils that had been lying in the ground for millions of years, right near where we looked at them. Park rangers have placed glass-topped boxes along the walkway, and the labels tell what ancient bones we're seeing. These are from eras after the extinction of the dinosaurs, when mammals had come into their own. There are fossils of long-extinct mammals related to present day cats, dogs, horses, and pigs. Each fossil represents an evolutionary dead end. They left no modern descendants, but they are related to existing species as distant cousins many times removed.

Nature is heartless in its wanton destruction of entire species, and always has been, even without our help. Now we're accelerating the process. We're a predator species that has wiped out countless other species by killing too many individuals for them to successfully reproduce in sufficient quantities to survive, as we almost did with the buffalo, and as we now seem to be doing with the wild salmon. We also alter their habitats, squeezing them out of house and home, or we produce wastes that poison them into oblivion.

Just because that's nature's way, doesn't make it right when we do it. We have big enough brains to be conscious of the deadly consequences of our conduct, so we should know better. And we're wiping out species at such an unprecedented rate that we reduce the biodiversity needed to keep whole communities of life thriving in ecological balance. We could well turn out to be the tipping-point species that turns the world into a desolate wasteland. Reading Jared Diamond's *Collapse* is what got me pondering whether we might be turning a fatal corner in our overly-successful run as a species.

We'll certainly get ours someday. Imagining that our own species will be spared from extinction is a theological fiction and an egocentric delusion. Judging by the way nature sits on its hands while species come and go, it seems we can no more prevent the eventual extinction of our own species than we can duck our own deaths. The only question is whether our species will survive long enough to leave descendant species before we all check out, or will humans too, become an evolutionary dead end? If we do evolve into another species, I'm guessing our distant descendants might return to smaller brains, seeing that nature's experiment in highly intelligent, manually dexterous, acquisitive mammals has some obvious flaws in the realm of over-consumption of resources.

When we came out of the trees and lost our fur, we became piss poor at surviving in the wild without acquiring the skins of other animals to keep us warm. So we used our handy ten digits to fashion tools to hunt them, and since we liked to eat their meat, we fashioned pots and baskets for carrying and cooking them. And from the early days, we've been fond of decorating ourselves with shells and feathers, even though jewelry has no direct functional value, so we had to find caves or build their equivalent to stash all our tools and pots and jewelry. Flash forward to mining diamonds and gold, with tremendous ecological and social harm, and to wiping out whole ecosystems to grow our monocultures of food, and to building monster houses to hold all the crap we've acquired. I suspect that evolving back toward our more physically hardy, less acquisitive ape roots might be our only chance as a species to leave descendants through the ages.

Personally, I don't find it depressing to contemplate the eventual demise of our species, for the same reasons that I don't brood over my own death. First, it's inevitable. Second, it hasn't happened yet. I'm here, breathing in and out and writing these words and enjoying the lingering taste on my tongue of some vanilla ice cream I just ate and waiting for my water to boil so I can savor a cup of tea on this chilly evening, on a day during which I saw winter's first snowflakes out the window. In the afternoon I napped, but it took time to fall asleep, because I lay there watching the snow fall in the New Hampshire woods, feeling as excited as a kid, remembering childhoods here, riding on my aluminum snow-coaster–the one I just found today out in the barn with my name painted on it in my own handwriting. I hung it on a nail out there so children in the Crooker clan can enjoy sliding out behind the house, just as I used to.

And today, up in the barn rafters I found Dad's old wooden skis with spring-style bindings and his initials, C.W.C., Charles Wescott Crooker. He enjoyed skiing right up until he died from a rare form of skin cancer called Merkel cell carcinoma. I brought his skis inside to decorate one wall of the family farmhouse. There's no sense fretting over my own death or my father's death or the death of our species. Life is good and will be good until it isn't.

◇◇◇◇◇

Chapter Eleven

After leaving Badlands National Park, I drove east across South Dakota as far as the Missouri River where I found an inviting campground on a rolling green hillside on a bluff above the river. I knew I was out of the arid West and into the Midwest because of my tent stakes. Instead of resisting the hammer in hard-packed soil, or sliding too easily into shifting sand, the tent stakes lodged with satisfying firmness in moist loam.

I had lost an hour when I crossed a time zone, so I decided to eat dinner in a local restaurant called Al's Oasis in Oacam, South Dakota, instead of taking time to cook in the campground. The meal involved a hunk of meatloaf and a mound of mashed potatoes because I had arrived at that part of our country. Never buck the local cuisine. They cook best what they like to eat, so I usually go with the flow.

The other patrons were middle Americans raised on middle American food and, at least two of them, on middle American fundamentalism. The husband had a swept-over-the-baldspot hairdo reminiscent of a televangelist. The slim, prim wife was dressed in a beige, structured suit; the kind that keeps its own shape, obscuring the contours of the body inside. She had the short, tightly curled hair typical of many midwestern ladies, who often resemble sheared sheep or clipped poodles. Two young waitresses, who apparently knew this couple, stood attentively by their table. The waitresses were about high school age, and they treated their elders with deference bordering on obsequiousness.

The woman was holding forth as if preaching to a

congregation while the girls nodded their silent agreement. She was exhorting these girls to live well. She warned them, "Your tongue is the most evil part of your body." It must have sounded so good to her that she repeated it. "Your tongue is the most evil part of your body." I suppose she was taking exception to the fundamentalist view that the genitals are the number one offenders, but I'm guessing this sanctimonious woman would have ranked the genitals as close runners up in an evil-parts-of-the-body contest. I, myself, have never thought to divide my body into good and evil parts. I've always assumed it's all one package. Maybe I should reconsider. Has my big toe been up to no good lately? How does my elbow fare in the eyes of the Lord?

It was not far from here, in a roadside restroom, that I picked up a pamphlet titled, "The Flag I Love." The words are printed over a red, white, and blue photo of a flag fluttering in the wind. The pamphlet is published, not by a veterans' organization, not by a military families' support group—none of that. It is published by Good News Publishers and distributed by a Baptist church. The pamphlet tells how we are stained by sin that can only be washed away by the blood of Jesus Christ, but that our flag shines brightly, "uncorrupted by any dark stain."

This pamphlet is an example of what I refer to as the Yankee-Doodle/Jesus Christ mix-up, with the U.S. flag taken hostage by a segment of Christian believers and boosted to the level of a religious icon. Have these folks never heard of the First Amendment—you know—separation of church and state? I've traveled enough now to reach the conclusion that confusing Yankee-Doodle for Jesus Christ is pandemic throughout our country.

I'm not a big fan of flags, because we should start paying more attention to our interconnected world, but I resent the hijacking of the U.S. flag for religious purposes. Hey, buddy, give me back my flag. It's mine too. It belongs to atheists and agnostics, Jews and Muslims, Buddhists and Hindus. It belongs to Native Americans and Chicanos, to African-Americans and Asian-Americans. It belongs to nudists and vegans and the spiritually non-aligned. It belongs to tree huggers and whale watchers and NPR listeners. It even belongs to all the guys in prison. Watch out, or I'll send Bubba to take back our flag.

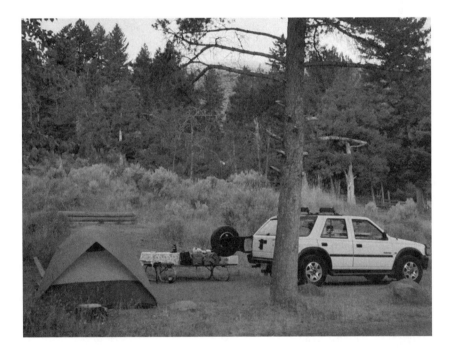

That night, alone in my tent, my mind traveled far from the Missouri River, far from meatloaf and gravy, and a world away from poodle-haired evangelists. I enjoyed a short story from a collection of stories by the Russian writer, Anton Chekhov. I have been reading one each night before sleeping. They are short enough that I can read them without wearing out the batteries in my camping lantern. *Selected Stories* was given to me by my friend, Peder, just before he left for Vietnam and before

I left for this trip. We often trade books on subjects of mutual interest, but I had never mentioned Chekhov. He either guessed I would like it, or was sharing what he enjoys, but it has been a delightful surprise. Thanks, Peder.

Chekhov is a joy to read, even though I must read the stories in translation. He's concise, precise, subtle, and a great observer of the rural Russian soul, with a Twain-like knack for a good twist at story's end. That night I read a perfectly structured, three-page story called, "The Decoration," in which a rural schoolteacher named Pustiakov begs to borrow a prestigious military medal from a friend so he can wear it to a party to impress the guests, especially the young ladies. When he sees a colleague at the same party who will spot the ruse, he must go through contortions to hide the medal throughout the dinner. When the colleague is asked to pass a platter of food, his coat falls open, and Pustiakov sees that the colleague has also been hiding a borrowed medal, except his friend's medal is of higher rank. Our protagonist is then able to display his own without fear of being outed as a fraud, and his only regret is that he hadn't chosen a higher rank for himself.

Goodnight, Peder. I hope you are enjoying Vietnam. Goodnight, televangelists. Keep enjoying Oacam, South Dakata. Goodnight, Chekhov, wherever you may be. Oh, and goodnight Lewis and Clark. I hope you enjoyed your trip past here on the Missouri River down the hill below where my tent is pitched. It's such a big and varied world. How could anybody ever be bored?

Now I'm cruising east on I-90, gobbling up miles of South Dakota on my way toward Minnesota. I'm listening to various National Public Radio stations. When I get out of range of one station, I hit the search button, and a different NPR station comes on with the same broadcast, so I hardly miss a beat. One NPR station out of Sioux City, South Dakota, plays great swing jazz. I tap my fingers on the steering wheel while listening to the likes of Tommy Dorsey, the Andrews Sisters, and Cab Calloway.

When I hear swing, I regret being born in the wrong era. Gotta love the boogie woogie bugle boy from company B. And did you know that the jim, jam, jump and the jumpin' jive makes you like your eggs on the Jersey side? It's true. It also makes you nine foot tall when you're four foot wide. Not only that, it makes you hep-hep on the mellow side. Give me some of that jim, jam, jump. I wanna jitterbug.

There's a great dance revival of Lindy Hop (a.k.a. jitterbug) going on in Portland, Oregon. Before anemia stole my energy, I would go out often and Lindy to my heart's content. I told my niece Elizabeth that the reason I like to Lindy is that when the boys fling you in the air, your underpants show. Elizabeth, who knows me well, said, "Aunt Connie. Be sure you're wearing some."

Soon after crossing into Minnesota, I saw a sign for the Pipestone National Monument. My parks pass made squealing noises in my wallet. It wanted to come out and play. I had never heard of Pipestone, so I checked my AAA guidebook, and Pipestone was marked with a gemstone, meaning it's worth seeing. It was thirty miles north, but that made a welcome break from freeway driving, so I headed north on fine, straight roads through rolling corn fields with cozy farms dotted here and there.

Pipestone is a smooth, red stone made of clay which has been compressed underground under subsequent layers of sandy rock, after being deposited in ancient bodies of water. Indians from different tribes all used it to make pipes for their smoking ceremonies. Pipestone National Monument is a site where the sought-after pipestone has been quarried for unknown centuries.

The tribes are said to have put aside warfare when they entered the sacred site of this shared resource. To enter the area, you pass three large boulders, which are either three maidens who guard the site, or three erratics (rocks deposited by melting glaciers far from their place of origin), depending on whether your source of information is tribal or scientific.

The Indians still quarry for their pipestone here, but the area is managed by the government. There are rangers on hand to answer questions, and there's a visitors center with a small museum, a workshop where the pipes are being made by Native American craftsmen, and a shop that sells the carved pipes. Outside, there's an active quarry that is being worked by tribal members.

I took a refreshing nature walk on the trails outside, and I chatted with a man working in one of the quarries. A pipestone quarry looks like a wide trench in the ground. This one was perhaps ten feet deep and four feet wide. The fellow working there told me that fall is the right season to get to the pipestone because, usually, the ground has dried out. But this year was rainy, so they've been spending all their time scooping mud out of the trench just to get down to the layer of red stone that lies deep in the earth. This man was not yet elderly, but getting along in years. He had worked the quarry most of his life, and had the attitude of a proprietor showing me his property. I guessed he had chosen this life because he liked the outdoors and being close to the soil. He didn't seem frustrated that the mud was slowing down this year's production. The pipestone would still be waiting when the mud dried out. No rush.

The park service's interpretive signs all emphasize the spiritual nature of this place and of the ceremonies in which the pipes are smoked. The tone is profoundly respectful. The stone is considered sacred and the act of smoking is spiritual because the smoke rises to heaven, carrying prayers.

I saw one of the Native Americans working the pipestone. He had examples around his workbench of finished products. Most were pipes, but there were other decorative objects also. One was a replica, in perfectly polished red stone, of the Starship Enterprise from Star Trek. I confirmed that's what it was, and we both had a good laugh. After all the pandering claptrap about spirituality written on the signs and in the pamphlets, I found this man's humor refreshing, as if he were saying, "The pipestone objects are sacred except when we say they aren't." Or maybe I'm wrong. Maybe the Enterprise is one more way of getting prayers up to heaven. Beam me up, Scotty.

In the museum were a few petroglyphs and pictographs that had been outside at this site, but that were now displayed indoors. A petroglyph is made by carving into the surface of rock, and a pictograph is made by painting onto the rock. There had been more of them outside, but souvenir hunters had stolen them. Some folks returned their stolen art to the museum, and that's why there is any left at all. The pictures may be small and sketchy, but these little goats and buffalo and stick figure men, some with headdresses, some holding arrows—all these pictures represent the messages and the dreams of native people from centuries in the past. Now they're reduced to a few remains, taken out of their original setting and context.

I lament the loss of petroglyphs and pictographs. Throughout the West they've been snatched by greedy folk, defaced by modern graffiti, buried underwater when dams have filled dry canyons with water, and worn away by the ravages of wind and weather.

The reason I'm passionate about petroglyphs and pictographs

is that they tell us more than other artifacts. When archaeologists dig up arrowheads or pottery, they use their detective-like skills to piece together whole cultures, and they tell us whether the people back then hunted or planted corn, and whether they lived in good-sized cities or scattered villages. But when we look at the art produced by ancient people, we glimpse their thoughts through dim and dusty time.

It's one thing when people create objects needed for survival, but it is another when they create art. Art is for communicating ideas. What they were communicating, and to whom, is subject to debate, but it is wonderful to know that the human mind has, for millennia, reached out to tell pictorial stories to others of our kind. We are the animal that has always expressed our hopes and dreams in pictures.

I have stood before similar images on rocks in Oregon, Utah, New Mexico, old Mexico, Arizona, Colorado, Puerto Rico—all over North America. I have read what others say about their meaning. The more I study this rock art, and read the theories of others, the more I realize how little anybody knows about its purpose. Even the tribes tell contradictory stories.

One famous image in Oregon, on a bluff beside the Columbia River, called "She Who Watches," has as many myths associated with her as there are tribes telling her story. I've seen her, and I'm not even convinced she's a woman. I think she might be a round-eared beaver with square little teeth. That's what occurred to me when I looked at her lovely, oval face, high above a river where beaver do, in fact, live.

Most archaeologists start with the assumption that these are primarily sacred images tied to ritual. They talk about shamanistic purposes and animal spirits. Some theorize that rock art is about praying for good hunting. I'm sure that's true for some of the art. But I have been persuaded by one author to think of some in a different light.

His theory is simple. Much rock art was an early form of writing. This theory was proposed by Lavan Martineau in a book called *The Rocks Begin to Speak*. The author is apparently not a well-accepted authority by others in the field, perhaps because he has no degree in art or archaeology. His claim to authority comes from a lifetime looking at rock art and pondering its meaning. I have a degree in art history, and this guy's theory makes sense to me. I'm not convinced of all the details of how he purports to "read" the messages on the rocks, but I'd bet my art history degree that he's on the right track.

Let's start way back. The prevailing theory is that Native Americans came from Asia. What culture has the most advanced form of pictographs ever devised? The Chinese. If the rudiments of Chinese pictographic writing had been in the works twelve thousand years ago, the concept would have traveled with the people who came across the northern land bridge to this continent.

Our modern western alphabet is based on phonetics. Each letter represents a sound, and when we stitch several letters together, they spell the sound of the spoken word. The Chinese alphabet consists of pictures that represent ideas, words, and thoughts. That's why they need thousands of characters to tell a story. Each word or idea gets its own separate picture. So the concept that a picture of three goats facing west would tell a different story than a picture of five buffalo facing east is not unfamiliar. You may not be talking about goats or buffalo at all. The animals could stand for something entirely different. They might be a form of writing—a set of symbols used to represent ideas.

Martineau suggests that some of these pictures express things like instructions to others who pass this way. For example, a set of symbols on a rock near a well-used trail might say, "If you go around behind these rocks, and then walk east to the tall pines, you'll find a water hole, but only in the springtime." If this theory is correct, then not all the rock art has shamanistic purposes. Some of it would be the equivalent of us putting up a sign that says, "Next exit, McDonald's."

I discussed this with a park ranger at Pipestone who was in agreement. He related an example of the plausibility of the communicative aspect of early Native American art. He said he'd seen a buffalo skin that was decorated with a spiral. Each year a symbol was added to the spiral's time line to signify that year's most important event. It was an example of a written history in pictorial form.

Several of the images at Pipestone's museum astonished me because I had seen them before. I saw them in far-off southern Utah. I was looking at figures with bodies shaped like upside-down triangles–wide at the shoulders and pointed at the bottom, where two stick-figure legs begin. The triangle would represent the area from shoulders to groin. Stick-figure arms go out from the points of the shoulders. The head is a simple circle. One character holds a tomahawk-shaped object and another holds a curvy, snake-like object. I swear I saw similar figures on rocks in southern Utah.

Maybe the triangular-body tribes traveled a long way to get their pipestone, or maybe the style of drawing was transmitted from tribe to tribe across the country, or maybe the people who had lived here later migrated to Utah. Not all rock art designs are similar, even in the same location. Different tribes pass through an area, sometimes hundreds or thousands of years apart, and their art varies. For example, right here at Pipestone, some figures have box-shaped bodies, and some have wide, straight bodies, where the sides of the torso continue to become the legs. So seeing this Utah style, triangular guy in Minnesota knocked me back.

The way some Native Americans used upside-down triangles to depict the body is something I've often pondered; often enough to come up with a theory. As usual, my theory is an unsubstantiated flight of fancy, but it has haunted me for years.

In 2002, I traveled with a small, hardy group of hikers to the Maze District of the Canyonlands National Park in southeast Utah. To get there, we drove forever on dirt roads that are impassable when desert storms turn the road to slick mud. Then we hiked six-hundred feet down into the canyon. Then we hiked several miles along the canyon floor until we came to Horseshoe Canyon, the site of what is considered by many to be the premier Native American rock art in the nation. All this hiking was in the hot desert sun, where sun protection and plenty of water are mandatory.

Horseshoe Canyon has a smooth wall that hosts the art. The larger-than-life figures there are said to be at least 2,000 years old. They have been described as ghostly and haunting. Although I believe not all rock art is about shamanistic rituals, the art here is otherworldly. The remote location, far from any known Indian village, past or present, would have made an ideal destination for a spiritual pilgrimage. Something very special went on here a very long time ago. The hair on the back of my neck still tingles when I remember this place.

There is a cluster of large figures high up on the rock. The bodies are shaped like upside down triangles, but with a difference from the Pipestone stick figures. They have no arms or legs. The triangle is thin and elongated, top to bottom. A couple of the faces have large, bulbous eyes. That is unusual for rock art, and is one feature that makes some of these figures so hauntingly vivid.

If these represent humans, where are their feet? Where are their hands? It's not for lack of drawing skill that they were omitted—after all, several of the faces have eyes, and some of the bodies are decorated with geometric designs. The artists could certainly have drawn hands and feet if they thought them important.

I suspect hands and feet weren't depicted because these characters had none. They weren't meant to be people. I think they are spirit people made in the image of ... of what, exactly? That's the problem with this theory. What are they supposed to look like? Here was my first clue.

I stood next to one of my co-travelers who gazed at one of the panels of rock art—not the same panel where these figures were, but close by. She said exactly what I was thinking: "Why did they paint a parsnip up there?" A parsnip. Precisely. An elongated, upside-down triangle, tufted on top. No human features at all. A plant.

"Think, Connie, think," I said to myself. If these were part of shamanistic rituals, they probably used hallucinogens to achieve their visions. Some Native Americans still do, so their ancestors probably did. What kind of hallucinogenic plant looks like a parsnip?

We know there are tribes that have used psilocybin mushrooms to experience visions. But mushrooms look like mushrooms, not parsnips.

There are tribes that have incorporated the hallucinogenic cactus, peyote, into their rites. The Huichol Indians in Mexico still use peyote in their sacred rituals, and much of their unique and detailed art is inspired by the colorful visions they experience. In the United States, the Native American Church has been granted a federal exemption from controlled substances prohibitions so that they can use peyote in their religious ceremonies. But there's a problem. A peyote cactus looks like a circular clump of roundish bumps. Circles within a circle. Peyote buttons do not resemble a parsnip.

There are tribes that have used datura to experience the infinite. But datura is a large-leafed plant, not an upside-down triangle. Come on, Connie, think.

I went home from that desert adventure full of the idea that I was onto something, but I was unable to find the plant that matched my theory. If a parsnip-shaped, hallucinogenic plant grew in this region, then these spirit figures might represent the plant itself manifested as spirits or gods. It makes sense that the plant itself would be revered, because the ecstatic visions in which the worshiper feels a connection with God, and the plant that produces the visions might be seen as one-in-the-same. The plant they eat would be the god, much like the bread and wine that Christians eat are said to be the blood and body of Christ himself.

Once at home, I called an old friend from hippy days. We used to call him Peyote Pete. He was quite the proponent of the white, hippy version of the Indian vision quest. He had trafficked in more peyote buttons than probably any white person in history. (That was a long time ago. All the statutes of limitations have run, so drug enforcement agents, stop drooling. Besides, I changed his name to protect the guilty.) I said, "Hey, Pete. What does a peyote plant look like when it's growing? You know, the part underground."

He said, "It's kind of like a big, fat carrot."

Bingo.

I went online and Googled around and found a picture of a peyote root. It looks just like a parsnip, which itself looks like a big, fat carrot. Seen from the side, the underground part of the plant would look like a parsnip which is topped, above ground, with a round, button-encrusted cactus that could inspire the image of the god's head with bulbous, peyote-button eyes.

So that's the unsubstantiated theory I dreamed up. It would explain why a 2,000-year-old picture of a parsnip appears on a rock near parsnip-shaped gods. And, my theory has one other great advantage. Since I don't claim it is true, nobody can shoot holes in it.

All these reflections were spurred by one look at a few triangular-shaped stick figures on a rock, in a museum in Pipestone, Minnesota. I'm grateful to all the Indians who created art throughout the ages for whatever purpose they had in mind. I'm so glad to be alive to admire it and puzzle over it.

My trip to Utah in 2002 was important for another reason pertinent to this story. That is when I first noticed my vitiligo. I mentioned earlier that I have had vitiligo since 2002, but that even with yearly skin checks by a dermatologist, nobody in the medical world was alert to its implications. Doctors in general have not yet learned that a melanoma history plus the onset of vitiligo equals a recurrence of the melanoma.

The Utah adventure was a tour with a small group from Portland, Oregon. It was a city-sponsored recreation activity. We were guided by the marvelous outdoorsman, Doug Ironside, to off-the-beaten-track locales throughout southern Utah. We traveled in a City of Roses van, with all our camping gear lashed on top. We camped in primitive campsites with zero amenities and we hiked all day, every day. At night we shared cooking and clean-up, then we chatted and sang around the campfire. Every day I was transported to a desert-induced euphoria.

Sunlight bathes the desert, and I had to protect myself. Ever since the cancerous mole was removed from my back in

1990, I have always covered up in sunlight. An entire section of my closet is filled with long-sleeved, white shirts and long, white pants. I own an embarrassing number of broad-brimmed hats. So I roamed the Utah desert smeared with sunblock and covered in white.

One day during the Utah trip, as I was putting on sunblock, I noticed that I had white splotches on my arms and legs. I don't know whether they had come on gradually and I hadn't noticed them, or whether being out in the sun had suddenly triggered the vitiligo. But I was soon assured by my dermatologist that, although they know little about its cause, and although the loss of coloring from the skin is permanent, vitiligo is nothing to worry about.

I will say again, loud and clear, that if you know of anybody with a history of melanoma who is diagnosed with vitiligo, that person should run, not walk to the nearest melanoma oncologist. Both my East Coast and my West Coast melanoma oncologists tell me that vitiligo in a melanoma patient is a sign that the immune system is amping up to fight the disease. They each noticed the correlation, because they saw vitiligo develop as one of the frequent side effects of interleukin-2 treatments. Spread the word, please.

I got the vitiligo in 2002 and the recurrence of my melanoma was not diagnosed until 2008, when I was found to have two large tumors. Six years had elapsed. The only good news is that I lived without treatment for those six years when I should have been a goner. That must mean that my own body, even without treatment, knows something about keeping these nasty melanoma cells at bay. Thank you, immune system!

◇◇◇◇◇

Chapter Twelve

Interleukin-2. I have often said that I wouldn't wish it on my worst enemy. Well, maybe my worst ... Usually, when a doctor warns you of side effects, they are remote possibilities. It's the doctor's malpractice insurer that requires the cover-your-ass warnings. With interleukin-2, the doctor warns you of a long list of side effects that are certain to wallop you. I knew I was in for a rough ride. Here is an email I sent to friends and family just before going into the hospital for treatment:

September, 20, 2008: It has been a long, slow crawl out of the cave of abdominal surgery, but I'm up and running again, *sans* anemia, which was cured when they chopped the tumor off my small intestine. The tumor was shipped to France, but didn't qualify for the study. (Not fluent enough in French?) So I start a standard treatment this week for the inoperable melanoma in my chest.

Here are the gruesome details for those with strong stomachs: I get interleukin-2, a natural protein of the body. It is immunotherapy designed to stimulate the immune system. I'm hospitalized for about six days at Dartmouth Hitchcock in Lebanon, New Hampshire, starting Thursday, September 25. They inject me with the stuff fourteen times, eight hours apart and then monitor my reaction. They promise swelling, a drop in blood pressure, and red, itchy skin. It looks much like my liver and kidneys are failing, "but they aren't," says the doc, reassuringly. Oh. And I also can "get confused." They skip a dose if the symptoms are too hideous.

Then they send me home for about nine days, and just when I'm feeling better, I go back for another round. And maybe a third round later.

Crisp, fall weather has come to NH, and the leaves are turning their famous colors. I picked tart cooking apples at a neighbor's beautiful farmland yesterday, under blue skies with views of wooded hills. Pumpkins abound. We've spotted a bobcat, three bald eagles, and eleven loons recently. Life is a wondrous thing.

I gratefully accept all prayers, incantations, voodoo, and hocus pocus that any of you send my way.

Due to an early morning hospital check-in, I stayed the night at an inexpensive hostel for patients in Hanover, New Hampshire, right next to the venerable Dartmouth College campus. Upper Valley Hostel is designed for patients who go frequently to Dartmouth-Hitchcock for chemo, radiation, or other regular treatments, but who live too far away to drive each day. The building is a lovely, remodeled private home with sixteen single beds in eight bedrooms on three floors. There is a common kitchen and living room.

The hostel is a godsend. A flock of volunteers stock the refrigerator with food, and deliver home-baked goodies. A florist donates fresh flowers. A bakery donates bread. Hand-knit afghans cover the beds. Nothing is overlooked to make the place feel homey.

I have fond memories of breakfast with the other patients. The hostel provided cereal, hot oatmeal, toast, fruit–whatever you might want to fix for yourself. I sat in the sunny dining area and began to talk with patients who were enduring grueling treatments for months at a time. They were grateful to talk with other patients who were teetering on the brink. Most late-stage patients keep a stiff-upper-lip around friends and family, so it is a relief for us to be surrounded by others who are looking death in the eye. Unlike other social settings, where patients tend to hold back information about their dire circumstances, here, at Upper Valley Hostel, we talked freely and frankly.

The night before, in my comfortable bed at the hostel, I had Teddy to clutch. In the morning, I was embraced by these determined, uncomplaining fellow travelers. I don't remember a single name, and only vaguely recall the faces. But I am grateful they were there that morning when I needed others to carry my fear in their hearts.

After breakfast, I had time for a walk before Mom and Frank came for me. They had booked a nearby bed and breakfast for the week, so they could visit me daily. Still in slow motion more than six weeks after my surgery, I walked my mincing walk around the spacious campus of Dartmouth College, watching the oh-so-young students on their bicycles and on foot, hustling and bustling. They had their whole lives ahead of them. If they were like I was in college, they had no idea where their lives and careers would take them. Even if they had plans, many would be buffeted by life into unexpected directions. I wanted to embrace them all and tell them to study enthusiastically and to choose careers they love and to enjoy life's roller-coaster ride and to make sweaty, bone-crunching love at every chance.

It was late September and the leaves were starting to turn. I thought of the lyrics to *September Song.* "The days dwindle down to a precious few." I thought, is this what it's like to be an old person, at the end of life, looking with envy at the young? But I'm not that old. It's not fair, dammit!

I returned to the hostel, and soon Mom and Frank came and took me to the hospital. I wish I could relate what happened in an orderly sequence, but that's impossible. The memory of my treatments is like the memory of a tumultuous dream. It comes back in snatches, all jumbled. I had two hospitalizations for IL-2. This first one was at the end of September in 2008. The second was in mid-October. Both times I was in the same room, and what happened there seems like something that happened in another lifetime to a different person.

I remember clearly what happened between the two treatments. I was so traumatized by the first round that I couldn't imagine voluntarily returning for the second. I have represented clients in criminal cases who have been ordered by a judge to turn themselves in to start serving a jail sentence on a certain date. I always wondered how they could walk into a cage where they are stripped of all control over life. Now I know that turning myself into jail would be a snap compared to going back for more IL-2. It was so close to impossible, it almost didn't happen. I was desperate for help.

I called the doctor's office and asked whether there was a support group for IL-2 patients. Not just any cancer support group. I needed to talk to others who had allowed this vision of hell to engulf them. There was no such group. Not enough people get this treatment for there to be a group.

Then I got a call back from the doctor's office. There was an IL-2 patient of Dr. Ernstoff's who was willing to talk with me. Franklin had gone through IL-2 treatments eight years prior. They gave me his phone number in Vermont. I wept with relief.

I called Franklin and he was happy to talk with me. We talked for over an hour. I suspected it was purging for him to describe the treatments he'd suffered through, because who but another IL-2 patient would be interested in hearing the gory details? Like combat veterans who refuse to discuss war, I imagine that most IL-2 patients lock the trauma in a mental closet and move on.

Franklin is a therapist with a kind and reassuring voice. He had indeed lived eight years past when everyone expected him to die, himself included. He thought his chance of survival was slim to none. He was ready to die.

He said, "I have nothing good to say about IL-2, except that I'm still here." It was the worst experience of his life. He got violently sick. His skin was one big rash. He puffed up like the Michelin tire man. Hallucinations haunted him. He vomited so much and so often he thought his stomach would come out his mouth. His blood pressure dropped so far that they transferred him to the intensive care unit. He almost died there. He can't remember how many days he spent in the ICU. It's all a blur to him now.

Before his treatments he had been a long-distance runner. After his treatments, he struggled to regain physical fitness. It took him a full year to regain any semblance of energy. He would go to the gym and never know whether he could get a good workout, or whether he would be sapped of energy. The waves of fatigue came in unpredictable cycles. He felt guilty trying to work out when he was so tired, because he felt he was bringing bad energy into the gym.

Now he is back to enjoying life and exercise. He is a practitioner of a Hawaiian massage technique called Lomi Lomi, and also of the healing method called Reiki. He sucks up health at every chance.

Knowing that somebody else lived through this treatment was good news. It was thrilling that Franklin had been enjoying years of life after treatment. It gave me hope. I can never thank him enough for sharing his IL-2 experience with me. It's the only way I could possibly have mustered the courage to go back for more.

At each of the two hospitalizations, the morning of check-in began with a surgical procedure. Because they would intravenously administer so many treatments, I needed to have a port installed in an artery in my neck instead of dripping chemical cocktails into the smaller veins of the arm. To put the port in, they first injected happy juice that made me unaware of the invasion. I vaguely remember kind people and a pleasant drifting feeling.

The port later caused problems when it clogged up and blocked the flow of fluids. The nurses constantly flushed it with the medical equivalent of Drano, but sometimes that wasn't enough. They discussed whether to have it reinserted surgically. I don't recall whether my clogged port reached crisis level or not. I'm dimly aware that keeping the darn thing open was a big deal, and it made the staff frustrated and grouchy.

Some of my memories of my IL-2 treatments I pieced together with help from my mother and my stepfather, Frank. They both sat at my bedside for hours each day. When I asked my mother whether she would help me remember these times, I gave her a chance to bow out, because I know it was tough on her to watch her child go through this. She agreed to talk about it, but Frank told me later that bringing back the memories disturbed her so much that she lost sleep and her digestion went haywire.

She tells me that she and Frank learned to time their hospital visits. When I was first given an IL-2 injection, it would render me unable to interact. I would nap. I would toss and turn. I might be awake, but with no interest in talking. As the eight-hour cycle passed before the next injection, I would regain some of my mental and physical capacities. Mom and Frank would try to visit me late in the cycle. Occasionally I was able to play Scrabble with Frank, but mostly we chatted or they sat and read while I rested.

I was on a special ward in a room that the staff tried to keep sterile. People had to leave their coats outside, and I couldn't receive flowers. The number of staff that constantly cycled through the room was greater than during my post-surgery care. It was the hawk patrol, forever tinkering with bags of fluid on my pain pole, and monitoring my life signs with a blood pressure cuff, a thermometer, and sometimes, when my blood pressure dropped too low, a portable heart monitor that had blinking lights like the console on the Starship Enterprise.

When I was alert, I walked around the ward, as I had done when recovering from surgery. I circled and circled, reading all the bulletin boards, peeking into rooms and glimpsing pale, bare butts poking through open hospital johnnies, or seeing a smiling young man, surrounded by a crowd of animated friends and family, or hearing somebody moaning in a dimly lit room where the blinds had been drawn.

Once I found a friend—a woman who was also walking in circles. She was also at crisis level, stripped of all hair from her chemo, with a staggering history of harsh treatments for whichever form of cancer was clobbering her. I think it was breast cancer. She was my friend because she was a tough, uncomplaining old bird who remembered lots of good times even during her treatments. Anybody with no hair, with chopped-off body parts, and with a prognosis of almost certain death, who still looks on the bright side, is my friend. We walked together several times, and I visited her in her room. When I went to look for her again, she was gone. I felt sad seeing her empty bed. I'm pretty sure they told me she went home. I hope she's doing well, wherever and whoever she is.

I actually enjoyed one stop that I sometimes made during my walk around the ward. There was a room with a refrigerator and cupboards that had snacks for us to raid at will. I took popsicles and dixie cups of ice cream whenever I had any hint of an appetite, which was seldom. The room seemed like a luxurious oasis to me–like a free hotel mini-bar. Free to me anyway. I'm sure my health insurer didn't consider it free food.

Speaking of my health insurer, they, of course tried their best to dump me. They decided that since I had spent so much time in New Hampshire, I was no longer an Oregon resident, which is a requirement for my coverage. Never mind that they were automatically deducting my premiums from my bank account every month. I had to prove that I owned my home in Oregon, that my car and drivers' license were registered there, and that I voted by absentee ballot in the Oregon elections. I had to do all this during the fall of 2008 when I was getting these treatments. Health insurers know how to hit you when you're down.

I can't imagine what would have happened if I had lost my coverage. I hope we get universal health care in this country, and that any new system isn't as botched as what we've got. This is one subject on which, uncharacteristically, I have no theory. How to implement universal health care is way over my head. But that it should be a public duty is as plain to me as our public duty to educate all our children.

Back to my not-so-free snacks. They'd placed no food restrictions on me, but food usually didn't tempt me. At times I was so nauseated, the mere thought of food set me to heaving. I remember feeling proud that I didn't puke as much as Franklin had. But it was misery when I did. I once crawled from my bed to try to reach the bathroom in time and didn't make it. I apologized for painting the floor with puke. The staff told me not to worry about it, but it bothered me that a stranger had to mop up my vomit. I felt humiliated.

To make matters worse, the south end of my digestive tract was also unhappy. 'Nuff said.

Retaining fluids was one of the troubling side effects. I

puffed up. My calves went straight down to my feet, swallowing my ankles. My stomach bloated, and my features disappeared in a puffed-balloon of a face. I gained over twenty pounds of fluid in six days. They had warned me to bring loose-fitting clothing to wear home. By the end, I looked as round and shapeless as the Pillsbury Dough Boy.

Itching skin was another side effect. Unsightly red blotches and scaly skin were bad enough, but head-to-toe unscratchable itches were intolerable. A nurse appeared with a mentholated cream, and smeared it all over my body. The menthol chilled me until I shivered, but it temporarily eased the misery. I used that cream at home for weeks after the treatments. For several weeks I stopped using soap when I showered, because no cleanser was mild enough for my raw skin. The skin eruptions went on for months. I scratched like a flea-bitten dog for the longest time.

About the confusion. In the hospital was a room with books, board games, children's toys, and also a computer terminal. When I was up to it, I could check my email. I think my cousin Steve visited me in that room, and I think his child played with the toys there, but I'm not sure if this is my memory, or if I created the memory after my mother told me that I had enjoyed a visit with them there. When she first told me that they had visited, I had no memory of having seen them. My mother was surprised that I could act alert and engaged and then not remember the events. It was the same with telephone calls. I learned to warn people not to be surprised if I didn't remember their calls. To this day, I notice blank spots in my memory. I have learned to write down everything I might need to recall.

The mental tricks went beyond forgetfulness. There was something about insects. They were in places they weren't supposed to be. I didn't mind when they moved up the walls, but when the insects crawled on the nurses, it bothered me. It didn't seem right that they would have insects on them. The insects puzzled me.

There was agitation. Sometimes, if it was mild enough, I could use my African rattle to calm myself, or I would watch the television channel that showed lovely nature pictures while soothing music played.

Once, a volunteer appeared with a small, Celtic harp. She asked if we would like her to play for us. We were delighted. She serenaded Mom, Frank, and me in the hospital room. She was real, unlike the insects. When she played, I was in a relatively clear part of the IL-2 cycle, and I remember traditional songs like, "Greensleeves." The gentle harp music laid down a bed of tranquility on which I could rest awhile.

One time, my agitation annoyed one of the nurses. I don't know what I said or did, but she scolded me for being out of control. I was furious. Hadn't anybody told her why I was out of control? Being scolded hurt my feelings. I told on her. I thought she was a bad nurse.

Once, I couldn't get a handle on the agitation. Deep breathing didn't help. My agitation turned to panic. I shivered and shook uncontrollably. I didn't know what to do. I saw my mother in her chair reading a book. I was desperate for help. I said, "Mom, can you sing me a lullaby?"

She put down her book. "What?"

"A lullaby. Can you sing one?"

She thought for a minute, remembering lyrics. Then she began to sing. I know this lullaby. I heard it when I was little. Somebody used to sing it to me. Mom? Or maybe Dad. I was tiny. I love this lullaby. It makes me feel better already.

Baby's boat's a silver moon
Sailing in the sky,
Sailing o'er a sea of sleep

While the clouds roll by.
Sail, baby, sail
Out upon the sea.
Only don't forget to sail
Back again to me.

I'm calmer now. The lullaby helped. Why is Mummy crying? I feel better. So, why is she crying? Oh, I get it. Those last words. She cried when she sang, "Only don't forget to sail back again to me." She thinks I'm sailing away from her. I won't sail away, Mummy. I'm still here. Don't cry. I'm better now. You made me feel better.

That was just one bout of agitation. There were many. One was worse than all the rest. There was no help for it. I was in bed. Mom was in her chair, reading. Frank was not in the room. I needed ... I needed ... what did I need? Something I couldn't get. I had to have it. I couldn't stay in the bed anymore. The bed was a bad place. I couldn't get comfortable. I had to leave the bed. The bed was torture. I had to get out instantly, any way I could.

Mom says I was thrashing–jerking my arms and legs. I remember one swift dive off the side of the bed. I rolled over and let my top half fall toward the floor. My legs were still on the bed, but I was on my way down.

Mom ran to catch me, yelling all the while. She says the room filled with people. The doctors must have been meeting in the hallway. They all rushed in at once. They hustled Mom out of the room. She doesn't know what they did with me.

I think they strapped me down. I'm not sure. Maybe they just put up the sides of the bed, but I couldn't move. I had a buzzer and I could call for help, but I had to stay put. It makes sense that they couldn't tranquilize me. My blood pressure was at rock bottom. I think they tied me in place. I remember worrying about how I would go to the bathroom. Why would I worry about that if I could get up and go there? I'm pretty sure they trussed me like a Thanksgiving turkey.

That's enough for now. I'm beginning to shake and shiver just remembering how it was. But I'm not in that room suffering. I'm in our New Hampshire farmhouse and the morning sun is streaming in the window beside me and cousin Ellen arrives tonight from Canada for Thanksgiving, and brother Chuck and his wife Adrian will drive up from Massachusetts, and Mom and Frank are coming over, and guess who's cooking. I'm the hostess. I'm preparing a huge meal of thanks. We'll eat and eat. There will be turkey and gravy, stuffing and cranberry sauce, and all the extras——potatoes, yams, dinner rolls with butter, pearl onions, broccoli, pickles, olives, and before the meal, fruit and nuts, chips and dips, and after the meal, pecan pie and blueberry pie with ice cream. And I won't forget the hot cider and the coffee. I'll use the old silverware and Great Grandma's dishes and a vintage lace tablecloth, and the centerpiece will feature rust-colored candles in turkey candleholders. And I'm going to eat some of everything and all the food will taste delicious and I will be the most thankful person in America this Thanksgiving. I won't be trussed like a Thanksgiving turkey. I'll be eating one.

Chapter Thirteen

After my leisurely tour of Pipestone National Monument, I pushed to rack up mileage on I-90 heading east through Minnesota. I felt the urge to hurry, so I neglected to pause and plan ahead for a campsite. The clouds thickened and turned to drizzle, then to rain. A pelting downpour obscured the scenery. Night fell and fatigue and hunger crept up on me. Through my rain-streaked windshield I spotted a sign that said, "Gas, food, lodging"–the type of place where clusters of chain businesses are placed conveniently beside the highway. I usually avoid these generic spots. I resent them for erasing America's colorful regional characteristics. But, like boxed macaroni and cheese, although bland, they are convenient in a pinch.

The turnoff I chose happened to be at Blue Earth, Minnesota. I turned at random into one of the parking lots to pause and check my AAA guidebook. I was feeling out of sorts. Fatigue, hunger, a touch of homesickness, and even loneliness dampened my enthusiasm. All these, plus the lack of a plan for the night's rest made me feel unhinged. The world took on a surreal aspect. Then I spotted, through my rain-streaked windshield, lit up with floodlights as if it were high renaissance art, a monumental, green statue. The unlikely vision made me queasy. I blinked and looked again. Strange but true, it was the Jolly Green Giant. Here's what my AAA guidebook said about it: "Blue Earth ... is home to the Jolly Green Giant, a statue more than 55 feet tall in Green Giant Park." The Jolly Green Giant has its own park.

The towering statue, glowing green in the darkness of a rainy night made me question what the hell I was doing there. That spurred me to wonder what the hell I was doing anywhere. I realized I needed a hot meal right away to regain my equilibrium. I grabbed a generic motel room and ate at a nondescript restaurant, feeling ashamed that I would have nothing juicy to report in my journal.

I found this Wikipedia entry on the Jolly Green Giant: "The Jolly Green Giant statue attracts over 10,000 visitors a year. In July 2007, the Blue Earth City Council approved space for a Green Giant memorabilia museum. Lowell Steen, of Blue Earth, has collected thousands of Green Giant items and will permanently loan them to the museum."

I didn't know there were thousands of Green Giant items, but good for Lowell Steen. Good for Blue Earth. Good for the Green Giant/Seneca Food Company. You have spared yourselves from the blight of the completely generic highway turnoff that I was complaining about. You've got something that nobody else in the world has. You've got the Jolly, ho, ho, ho, Green Giant.

The next morning, rain still pounded the pavement. I had lingered long enough in the western states that I chose to zip along the eastern highways. The rain gave me an excuse not to stop and sightsee. There is something pleasurable in the rhythm of long-distance driving, with my own thoughts as the closest companion. I drift into a reverie and fifty or sixty miles melt away without much effort on my part. There's calm in the ticking of windshield wipers, and the closed-in-a-bubble sense that comes when landscapes are erased by a grey veil of rain.

That morning, my reverie was marred by semis. I crossed Minnesota in a streaking downpour seeing only my windshield wipers and the ass-end of monster trucks that flung entire puddles at me, doubling the amount of water on my windshield. I hear Minnesota is a lovely state. Next time perhaps I'll see it.

At least I found good radio stations.

I listened to a Dvořák piece with layered strings so rich in unexpected harmonies and contrapuntal melodies that I was spellbound. Then, my eclectic tastes prevailing, I switched to a station with Mexican music.

I admire the folk art that non-famous Mexican musicians manage to get played on the radio. They enjoy their flash of fame, just as one-hit-wonder bands did in the U.S. in the fifties before musicians had to sell their souls to a big label to be heard.

These Mexican songs often have sly double meanings, where barnyard antics, especially those of roosters, stand in for good times in the sack. The rural poetry can be sweet and funny. But one song disturbed me because the lyricist neglected to write in metaphors, and the lyrics were bluntly crude. A growly-voiced man sang that he didn't want to be just friends. "I want to *meterme en tu cuerpo*," meaning literally, "I want to put myself in your body," with the "put" carrying a tone of force. A fair translation would be, "I want to shove it in you." I hoped this was not the beginning of a songwriting trend.

I switched stations and found classic country music characterized by simple and true lyrics that nail the human condition in one phrase. "I go walking after midnight, searchin' for you." Oh my god. There goes Patsy Cline wandering around by herself on a road in the pitch black, in the middle of the night, hoping to catch sight of her ex. How obsessed and lonely can you get?

I heard a newer country song in the same classic vein. A man is chastised by his wife for seeking money over honey, so he promises that from now on he'll "light the bedroom candles and unplug the phone." Simple, but true-to-life stories make for good songwriting.

I saw that overworked man at a rest area, walking from his

car to the rest rooms. He was a stiff-backed, beefy farmer. The rain poured down, and he held a flowered umbrella tilted, not over himself, but to one side, over his biscuits-and-gravy-fed, butterball wife, who pressed to his side, clinging to his arm with both her hands. There was not one hair-breadth of space between them as he provided her shelter from the rain. Sweet.

By midday, I reached the Mississippi River at the Minnesota/Wisconsin border. The mighty Mississippi is mythic. It sets me dreaming of lazy days drifting on a raft with Huck Finn and Jim. It makes me want to hang out with riverboat gamblers on sternwheelers with Dixieland jazz bands. It reminds me of pre-rail, major shipping routes.

Fast-forward to modern times. I think of how the Mississippi carries enough nitrogen from nitrate fertilizers in the farm states into the Gulf of Mexico to create one of the world's largest dead zones—a place where fish can't live because there's not enough oxygen in the water. There's not enough oxygen because the nitrogen is gobbled up by algae that thrives, and grows. When it dies, it decays, which uses up oxygen. Although other causes may contribute to the oxygen depletion in the dead zone, the general consensus is that farming methods must be changed to keep from wiping out the Gulf's fishing industry.

Corn, the Midwest's main crop, is the biggest offender because its capacity for nitrogen uptake from the soil is so inefficient. Soybeans do better at nitrogen uptake, so alternating corn with soy helps some, but unless corn can be genetically engineered to take up more nitrogen, the environment is in trouble. Lowering our dependence on corn would help, but corn is the main feed for cattle, plus it is used in a huge percentage of the processed foods in the grocery stores. Sorry for the bad news. Don't shoot the messenger.

In spite of this, the Mississippi River is a lovely sight. The riverside is lushly wooded on the bordering bluffs. The broad, green leaves of deciduous trees make me feel like I'm getting closer to the forests of New Hampshire.

New Hampshire is thick with deciduous forests. In fact, it is one of the few areas in the world that is more forested than it was a century ago, back when farmers had cleared most of its arable land. Now bear, moose, and beaver are all back in business. Wild turkeys are everywhere. I've seen more bears in my own backyard than I saw in Yellowstone. I've even seen bobcats there. New Hampshire's ecological revival is heralded as an example of how we can turn things around, but I'm not convinced the change is permanent.

New Hampshire was an area where, in the 1800's, farmers reluctantly settled. Reluctantly, because the glacier-scoured land is rocky beyond belief. Much of the state is hilly to mountainous, and the growing season is short. Later in the 1800's, when the Midwest opened up for farming, with its flat, rich farmlands and its longer growing seasons, all the New Hampshire farmers with any sense headed west, never to return.

Now, New Hampshire's main industry is tourism, so the incentive is to keep things looking wild. Each autumn, hordes of "leaf peepers" arrive in tour buses just to see the fall foliage paint the entire countryside in blazing reds and oranges. But I predict that, if a growing population spurs the need to farm every farmable acre, we'll see the forests disappear again.

Could population pressures do that? When I was born, in 1946, there were three billion people in the world. That was up from one billion in about 1800. In my lifetime, the world population has more than doubled from three billion to over seven billion. More than doubled. Think about it. It took the whole history of life on earth to get to three billion humans. Then it took only sixty years to more than double that. That's huge!

An organization called Negative Population Growth claims (admittedly, not without controversy) that scientists put the optimal population for the United States at 150 million people. We already have over 300 million. NPG claims that those scientists also put the optimum size for world population at three billion. We've more than doubled that, too. I'm not vouching for this organization, but if these figures are close to valid, we're already in deep doo doo, population-wise. Even if this organization is wrong, we're clearly heading for trouble.

Our small orb hosts seven billion and counting of large, acquisitive mammals all needing at least some food, water, clean air, clothing, and shelter, with many of us gobbling up more than our share. So, could worldwide hunger cause New Hampshire to lose all its forests to farms again? Just asking.

Although I'm alert to the harm from overpopulation, I don't fret much about it. I have trained myself to get worked up over only those problems I have some chance of fixing, and I've already done my part to ease overpopulation. I neglected to breed. I award myself enviro-credits in a personal cap-and-trade scheme of my own invention that applies only to me. Since I failed to give birth to my allotted number of consumers, each of whom would require a house, television, computer, car and so on, I calculate that I can, without guilt, occasionally toss a recyclable container in with the household trash. So I don't brood over the pending overpopulation crisis. Someone else can fix this mess.

Now back to the Mississippi. The river's wooded banks reminded me of New Hampshire, but I saw lovely birds that we don't see that far north. Gleaming white egrets were wading in the marshes beside the Mississippi. Although we humans almost wiped them out in the era when we made ladies' hats from their lush feathers, fashions changed in the nick of time for the lovely birds. With their sinuous S-shaped necks and their dainty steps on long, spindly legs, they are one of nature's many wonders. Their legs are designed to look like twigs that fool fish into swimming right up to them. That's why they stand still for so long in the water. Then all they have to do is thrust their beaks in and grab a snack.

When I say "designed," I am speaking poetically and not scientifically. Creationists ask how nature can produce such marvelous designs without a designer. They can't believe that nature's dice-rolling is capable of producing such marvels. Believe it. It is precisely because nature is such a rough and tumble place that any newer and better model that chances to come along gets the advantage in the game of survival. When a so-called intelligent designer gets in the business of tinkering with evolution, as humans do when we breed animals, we produce freaks of nature, like turkeys that taste good but are too dumb to come in out of the rain. And Chihuahuas. I wouldn't want any intelligent designer mucking up our system of evolution. The system we have works just fine.

Having turned south at La Crosse, Wisconsin, I followed the Mississippi on one of AAA's scenic routes, first on the Wisconsin side, then, crossing back over to the west, on the Iowa side. As I traveled south, the sun came out. There. That's better. The world looks all sparkly new.

I enjoyed the rolling hills of Iowa, dotted with neat farms. I must admit, when I see a barn silhouetted on a ridge with fields spread around it, I romanticize the rural life. I picture Timmy's mom in her ruffled apron, serving home-baked bread and fresh-churned butter while Lassie runs home to grab help for Timmy, who just fell down the well. I'm not very realistic about farm life, since I know so little about it.

I have fun traveling with my friend Carol, who owns the

ranch in Wallowa, Oregon where Nora, Carol's daughter, slaughtered the goat. Carol can glance at any farm as we pass by, and tell how prosperous it is, what kind of crops and livestock they specialize in, and whether the farmer is a good steward of the land or a useless drunkard. All I see are pretty pictures on a calendar. Sorry. I hope all these people living on Iowa's farmland near the Mississippi are as contented as I pictured them. They feed all of us, and I'm grateful for their dedication.

The next day was another long day of driving, with all of it on multi-lane highways. Not my favorite style, but I had talked to cousin Ellen, and I was getting anxious to see her soon on my way through London, Ontario.

It was obvious by the traffic that I was entering the populous East. Driving around Gary, Indiana is not for the faint of heart. The traffic is like a herd of restless beasts, never happy with the lane in which they are traveling. The highway is a maze of on and off ramps, a forest of route number signs, and in the midst of it all, construction. The interstate was riddled with miles of single-lane driving due to repairs. It seems they threw a blizzard of federal stimulus money at "shovel ready" projects that had been put off for years, and they were now doing them all at once. Lucky me to witness, first-hand, our alleged economic recovery.

Looking for a campground that night was as frustrating as that day's drive. I had looked forward to an idyllic evening camped on the eastern shore of Lake Michigan, but campgrounds eluded me. In spite of maps, guidebooks, and cell phone calls to likely places, trying to locate a campsite was like a dream where you urgently need to reach a goal, but obstacles constantly deter you. After useless side trips to non-existent camping spots, well after dark, late at night, I turned in at a motel.

So I had one disappointing day out of the whole trip. So

what? By my standards, any day I'm not having my gut chopped in two, and not having my veins flooded with interleukin-2, and not having my chest bombarded with radioactivity–that's a good day. One thing cancer has done for me–it has reset the pleasure bar. Especially the IL-2. Especially that. To call IL-2 hell on earth is a euphemism.

◇◇◇◇◇

Chapter Fourteen

When I was writing before about my interleukin-2 treatments, I got shaky, felt sick, and had to stop. Now I can face those memories again. The treatment goal was to try for at least fourteen IL-2 injections during each hospitalization. They space each injection eight hours apart. When I got too wiggy, or when my vital signs turned less than vital, they would skip an injection. They managed to get nine injections in me during the first hospitalization, which was in September of 2008. The second time, in October, I tolerated only seven, but they considered both treatment sessions to be successful. Apparently few patients tolerate the full schedule of interleukin-2.

During my second hospital stay, my plummeting blood pressure caused a crisis. I mercifully don't remember much about it. I know I ended up in the intensive care unit. I recall a rush of personnel huddling around my bed and a portable heart-monitoring machine. I remember somebody asking me how I would like it if they stopped the IL-2. I liked it just fine, but worried about whether I had flunked out. I knew I needed at least a minimum number of treatments, and I would have toughed it out if my body would only cooperate, but my systems were shutting down.

I don't remember the days passing in the intensive care unit, but the medical record says I spent three days there. I recall no dramatic treatments. The report says I was given "pressors," to counteract my low blood pressure. I remember no feelings about being there. From my point of view today, I didn't feel sick, afraid, anxious, or anything. That's the point. I didn't feel anything. I don't remember leaving the bed. I must have stayed there until I could get up again.

I do remember that when they told me I could go home, my sister, Catherine, was there. She went to a pharmacy to fill my prescriptions and left behind her precious Red Sox baseball cap. If anybody at Dartmouth-Hitchcock finds Cathy's Red Sox cap, could you please return it? She's a gung-ho fan. It bothers me that she got so distracted about me that she left her favorite hat. Strange. I don't remember nearly dying, but I remember feeling bad about her lost baseball cap.

It was October 19th of 2008 that we returned to Mom and Frank's house, where I spent days lying on their couch. The IL-2's aftereffects were gruesome. I had gained over twenty pounds of fluid, and I looked ridiculous, but I was beyond vanity. I simply wanted to feel less bloated and disconnected. I took pills to speed up the passing of all that fluid, so I wore a trail to the bathroom.

My skin itched from the top of my head to the soles of my feet. I broke out in red blotches. The itching attacked suddenly in intolerable waves of impossible-to-calm torture. I slathered on a strongly mentholated cream, which helped temporarily, but it left me chilled.

I could only wear one item of clothing. It was a silky kimono that didn't bind anywhere. Anything else inflamed my burning skin.

The unpleasant combination of diarrhea and gas were (and still are) a problem. I still take medicine to tame the diarrhea.

Fatigue was a problem, and still is. I would feel like I was gaining ground, only to be ambushed by a dire need to lie down. I didn't dare wander very far from home for the first week. It was almost a year before I could go without an afternoon nap.

Here's a list of IL-2's side effects that I reported to my doctor:

◊ Teeth-chattering chills
◊ 103-degree fever
◊ Red, puffy skin
◊ Hive-like, itchy spots
◊ Dry mouth
◊ Cracked lips
◊ Diarrhea
◊ Itchy anus
◊ Agitation and fearfulness:
◊ Shortness of breath made me fear I couldn't breathe. In the hospital, I asked for and got oxygen.
◊ Visual and mental distortions:
◊ Green, bar-like lights by hospital door and TV
◊ Spider cracks on TV
◊ Black flies buzzing around
◊ Rushing animals at periphery
◊ Greeted sister and was glad she stayed in room next to mine, until I realized she wouldn't be coming for two more weeks.
◊ No memory of many phone calls.
◊ Loss of balance:
◊ I had a bell by my bed to wake parents to monitor my bathroom use in the night in case I fell.
◊ 22-pound weight gain
◊ Loss of appetite
◊ Inability to concentrate:
◊ Hard to find the computer keys to send emails
◊ Couldn't read
◊ Sleepiness alternating with agitated sleeplessness
◊ Couldn't bend to put on shoes
◊ Dry, stuffed nose
◊ Bloody mucous

◊ Parents had to monitor meds, use of scale, all aftercare instructions
◊ Wildly fluctuating food tastes:
◊ Popsicles and Cheeze-It crackers taste good. Vegetables, bad.
◊ Splitting headaches
◊ Nightmares
◊ Stitches in side
◊ Lower back pain

This list doesn't include one humiliating side effect that I reported to the doctor, but which I'm reluctant to write about. But I promised to tell the truth, and if this information could help even one other woman who must suffer through IL-2 treatments, then it should be told. IL-2 can weaken bladder control, which, in my case, didn't surface often, but it came on, to my great inconvenience, at the moment of the release of tension during an orgasm. Since I am clearly single, you might ask yourselves, to what orgasm is she referring? Just because I'm single doesn't mean that my itches need not be scratched. I discovered that, for about six months after IL-2, it was only safe to reach orgasm while seated on the toilet. I know that this would cause my niece, Elizabeth, to block her ears and holler, "*Too much information, Aunt Connie*," but I want to assure any woman who might be ambushed by this humiliation that it is only temporary. In time, my bladder control returned, and orgasms are sweet again.

In the month following my second round of IL-2, I worked to pull myself together as much as possible. I returned to exercise classes, modifying the routines to do what little I could. I soon moved from Mom and Frank's house back into the farmhouse and was able to stay there on my own, but many of the side effects lingered. I would scratch myself to sleep each night for weeks.

Enough of such misery. Let's get back on the road, back to the eastern shore of Lake Michigan. I had endured hideous traffic through numerous construction zones near Gary, Indiana. I had passed an area thick with appallingly tasteless billboard blight. On top of that, the lovely lakeside campground I longed for eluded me. But after enduring IL-2, a bit of highway tedium is a minor frustration.

I was exhausted and needed rest. I found it in a nondescript motel. The man behind the desk, one Mr. Patel, was gracious and helpful. I was still hoping to camp, and he helped me call several campgrounds, but nobody answered. It was towards the end of the camping season, and campgrounds were apparently closed. Then Mr. Patel kindly offered me a sixty-dollar room for forty five. I gratefully accepted.

I settled into my room and phoned my mother in New Hampshire. Family news. Cousin Steve had surgery Thursday for rectal cancer at Dartmouth-Hitchcock, the same place where I had my interleukin-2 treatments the year before. She tells me that he'll be in there for at least eight days. That means he'll still be there when I pass through, so I will visit him. His father, my Uncle Bill, now in his late 80's, has diabetes that causes such bad sores on his leg that the doctors might have to amputate it. He can't drive to see his son in the hospital, so I will pick up Uncle Bill and take him to see cousin Steve.

Just last year Uncle Bill and Steve were visiting me in Dartmouth-Hitchcock, thinking it might be the last time they would see me. It will be strange returning there as the healthy one.

As children, cousin Steve was closer to my younger brother Chuck than to me. They were rambunctious, and it's open to question which led the other astray, but they were constantly up to no good. I seem to recall something about BB guns and a neighbor's windows. That sort of mischief.

Now Steve and I have a newly-formed bond. Cancer will do that. He emails me details of his treatments: his chemo and his surgery. His cancer is potentially tragic. He's almost sixty and has just married a beautiful Filipina in her twenties. They have a shiny new baby together, plus he is Daddy to her four-year-old girl. His charming, gracious wife is new to this country and to their marriage, and suddenly rectal cancer threatens to wreck it all. Steve remains optimistic in spite of his grueling ordeal.

It will be a pleasure to visit him, especially since I'm doing so well. My chances were close to zero, and look at me now. I can give him encouragement and hope.

Dartmouth-Hitchcock, cancer, and my family. There's been too much of that combo. Here's another biggie. That's where my father was treated for his fatal case of Merkel cell carcinoma, a skin cancer so rare that there was no standard treatment for it. Not knowing what else to do, the doctors winged it with random chemotherapy. Dad's cancer was discovered after it had spread to internal organs. He died less than one year after diagnosis.

I remember visiting him in his hospital room at Dartmouth-Hitchcock and bringing him a stuffed moose. I blew up a rubber glove and drew a rooster face on it with a pen—the inflated fingers make the rooster's coxcomb. I once wrote a short piece about seeing him in the hospital, and I described his head, balding from chemo, as looking like "a skull in the making." I hesitated to write those words because it seems wrong to picture a loved one as already dead. But a writer's duty is to tell the truth. When I saw my father shrinking and shriveling up in his hospital bed, that's what his head looked like. So I wrote the words. The article was published. A reader thanked me for writing "skull in the making." He told me that he thought the same thing on seeing a loved one near death and felt guilty for thinking that way. It relieved him to know he was not alone. We should never lie about death. Even our harshest words might help somebody, if only to recognize our common human bonds.

Nor should we always take death seriously. The Mexicans have a colorful tradition of laughing at death as part of their Day of the Dead ceremonies. They make skulls into candies for children. They dress up skeletons as pompous politicians or vainly attired ladies.

Back in Michigan, in the nondescript motel presided over by the kindly Mr. Patel, I enjoyed some humorous thoughts about death. In the morning, as I was picking up some continental breakfast in the lobby, I overheard Mr. Patel talking on the phone. He said, "He's not answering his phone. Would you like me to knock on his door for you?" Mr. Patel went off down the hallway.

My imagination went wild. I decided he would find a corpse there, and with luck it would be a murder, and cops and detectives would soon overrun the place. There might even be a mad serial killer on the loose. How fun.

It could happen. People sometimes die in motels. Once while visiting Mexico with my friend Carol–the friend who knows all about ranching–we were enjoying an evening at a charming hotel in Acapulco; one that clings to rustic simplicity in the midst of overblown resorts. We had been invited to dine on the oceanside deck, under the palms with Fito, the owner's son. Picture a lovely, romantic setting, complete with sunset over the ocean, plenty of fresh seafood, and gracious company.

Carol used to own a remote dude ranch in Oregon's Wallowa mountains. So she and Fito got talking about the trials and tribulations of running lodgings for guests. The subject turned to what must be done when a corpse inconveniently makes an appearance at your lodgings.

In Carol's case, the guest dropped dead while on a guided elk-hunting trip, far from the lodge. She explained how you must strap the body onto the horse, but not in the over-the-saddle position you see in cowboy movies, with arms down one side, and legs down the other. If you do, gooey, hot bile will spill out each end and needlessly burn the horse's legs. You must tie the corpse in a normal seated position, but only until you get near civilization. Then you wrap up the body and drape it over the saddle to meet conventional expectations. People will think it's corpse abuse to prop the guy up in the saddle. Who knew there's a right and wrong way to pack out a cadaver?

In Fito's case, he told us his guests consisted of a family that had included a grandmother until granny checked out. Permanently. So what does the family do? They take their dear *abuelita* and stretch her out on the hotel lawn and place a circle of votive candles around her, and they begin their mourning right then and there. So, the *velas* are flickering, and the family is gathered around praying to the Virgin and the Santo Niño. The other guests are passing by, looking dismayed while granny's getting ripe in the tropical heat. So Fito and his father kindly suggest that they would be happy to call the local funeral home to come and take care of the dearly departed. But no. The family is afraid that if a local mortician shows up, he'll bury granny locally, and that would never do. Mexicans will spend their last *peso* to get the body of a loved one back to the town of origin to be buried in the person's native soil.

The family didn't own a car, so what did they do? They rolled sweet *abuelita* inside a carpet and tied her in there, and placed her as excess baggage in the luggage compartment of a public bus that took them back to their town.

So, in this Michigan motel, I'm waiting for Mr. Patel to return with dramatic news for the wife that her husband died, but no such luck. I overheard him telling her that that her husband had slept through the ringing telephone. Likely story. I bet the husband was in there with three or four underage hookers of indistinct gender, too distracted to answer the phone.

After eating my not-so-continental breakfast–how European is a bowl of Cheerios?–it was time to hit the road, east across Michigan toward London, Ontario to visit cousin Ellen.

◇◇◇◇◇

Chapter Fifteen

It was late October, 2008 when the interleukin-2 treatments ended. My only job was to recover and to wait and see whether the treatments had helped to shrink the inoperable tumor in my chest. Not knowing whether I would live or die, I couldn't make plans. But living an unplanned life is not all bad. Here's part of an email I wrote to friends and family while still in medical limbo in New Hampshire:

> Nov 1, 2008: My life is unplanned and unscheduled. There's a kind of freedom to that. Don't you wish you could erase everything from your calendar and do whatever you wish? I still exercise as much as I'm able (I do the geriatric shuffle for about half a mile now), I go to an Italian class and I attend a stimulating weekly discussion group where we wax philosophic on a multitude of themes. Plus I have enjoyed blazing fall foliage and a backyard bobcat sighting. (Here, kitty kitty.) I marched in the Columbus Day parade with the Over the Hill Hikers and I won a ribbon for an antique quilt I entered in the town fair. Big doings in a small town.

Then in December of 2008, the first scan following the interleukin-2 treatments showed that the inoperable tumor in my chest had not grown. I knew not to celebrate wildly, but I felt I could safely switch my medical care back to Oregon. I said my thanks and good-byes to Dr. Ernstoff and returned to Portland. Here's how I reported it in an email:

December 7, 2008: This is to keep you informed that the doctor here in New Hampshire says I can go back to Oregon. I leave on Friday, December 12 with mixed feelings. This New Hampshire town has become dear to me, but my other home is calling.

The latest scan shows that the tumor in my chest has not grown. This is good news. It means the interleukin treatments are having at least some effect, or the tumor would be bigger by now. We had hoped for shrinkage, but will have to wait one more month for another scan, to see which way the tumor will go. I'll have that scan in Oregon on January 5, with any follow up treatments there.

In the meantime, I've got enough of my energy back that I'm ready for skiing on Mt. Hood, dancing, and enjoying Christmas with my West Coast friends and family.

I left for Oregon with hope that the stagnant tumor would shrink, mixed with dread that it might grow by the time of the next scan on January 5. I arrived at my home in Portland just as Portland got hammered by massive snowstorms that kept the city paralyzed for two weeks. Here's an emailed Christmas message I sent that year:

December 22, 2008: Here's how wild our weather is in Portland. We got four inches of snow last night on top of yesterday's eight inches on top of all last week's snow. I just saw a city snowplow stuck in deep snow near my house on one of our main roadways. His big, fat, chained-up tires kept spinning uselessly.

Now I'm watching a man with a stuck Jeep who is digging the snow away from his tires with his bare hands.

He looks like a dog digging in sand.

Now he's at the wheel and his tires are spinning in place. Now he's back out using a window scraper for a snow shovel. Good luck, buddy. Now a good Samaritan has stopped and they're talking and scratching their heads. Now the Samaritan is gone, and the man is sitting in his car with the engine running to stay warm. Now his tires spin some more. This is less than five minutes from downtown Portland. There is one lane where traffic moves along slowly, but those who turn off it are doomed.

Sequel: I took pity on the man and went out with my snow shovel. He dug for half an hour. He had pulled off because he'd lost visibility, so he'd blindly picked the deepest spot in the snow, and his whole frame was hung up on it. He finally rolled off down the road, where he will be spending the day working on the construction of a new wing on a hospital.

The snow is beautiful. I have food, movies, and a fireplace, and my power has stayed on, so far. It's getting light out now, so, after breakfast, I think I'll go out and do some city snowshoeing.

Please consider this my Christmas card since no way am I getting to the post office. Happy holidays!

The same day I sent that email, I did, indeed do some city snowshoeing. I lent my extra pair of snowshoes to my neighbor, Chris, and we were able to walk to the center of Portland without having to remove the snowshoes for bare pavement. There was none. There had been so much snow, people gave up shoveling the sidewalks. It thrilled me to see the city transformed by mounds of white and thrilled me more that I could get out and enjoy it. It had been only two months since my last IL-2 treatment, and I was doing a *Nanook of the North* imitation in the middle of the city. Of course it was tiring, and on the return trip from downtown, I could barely lift the snowshoes, but I made it. I came up with a new cliché to replace the one about life handing you lemons. When life hands you a snowstorm, go snowshoeing.

Not that all was peachy and rosy. I had become anxious to return from New Hampshire to Oregon so I could begin cleaning out my house. It felt like my time was limited, and I didn't want to burden my sister Catherine with sorting all my stuff after my death. But facing my possessions was overwhelming. I had little enthusiasm and even less energy for the project.

When I mentioned my efforts to Catherine, she said, "What are you doing?"

I said, "Cleaning out my house so you don't have to."

She said, "Leave it. It's just stuff. Use your time to dance and ski."

I was flooded with relief. I had little decision-making ability left after my treatments. It was a major chore to sort possessions. What stays? What goes? Who gets what? It was physically challenging to lift and stoop and pack and label. I gladly gave it up.

I did no Christmas shopping in 2008. All the gifts came from my drawers and closets—treasured possessions I wanted to pass on. A friend called and told me I had left a valuable handmade basket at a potluck, and that she still had it. I told her the background story of the lovely basket, and told her to keep it. Of all my friends, she would appreciate it most.

I surveyed my closet and decided that I would probably never go shopping again. I had enough clothing, shoes, hats, and purses to outlast me. I counted my bars of soap in the bathroom. I would never need to purchase more soap.

In early January, I got my next scan. The tumor was no longer stable. It was not shrinking. The tumor was growing. My deepest fear turned real. After all I'd been through, my last shreds of hope dissolved. I should have known. I could feel pain from the cancer, but had tried to minimize it. Although I had been gradually preparing to die, the reality of death's proximity was still a shock.

Ever since Thanksgiving of 2008, I had started to notice that it hurt to swallow. Food would sometimes stick in my throat, and I would have to wash it down with a drink of water. I learned to chew food to mush before swallowing. I learned to take tiny bites. By Christmas, eating was always painful. I worked to hide my pain from my sister and her family during that year's Christmas dinner.

Then, in early January I saw a picture of my throat taken by ultrasound. That shocking image is burned in my memory. My esophagus was blocked off with only a tiny passage open at one side. The tumor bulged into my throat and pushed my esophagus closed. No wonder it hurt to eat.

I went through a whirlwind round of medical appointments to explore options. They might remove the esophagus and surgically pull the stomach up to the throat. They might put in a stent—a rigid tube—to hold the esophagus open. They might put in a bypass feeding tube to funnel nutrition directly to the stomach. The tumor itself was not operable because it was in what one doctor called the "high-priced real estate" of my upper chest where its proximity to heart, lungs, and major blood vessels made surgery too risky.

The thought of a bypass feeding tube terrified me. I said, "You mean I would never eat food again?"

"That's right."

The doctor was calm and cool, delivering the news as if I'd be pleased that he had a solution for me. He even said, "Don't worry. We won't let you starve to death."

Never eating food. A living, breathing creature, wired to spend a good part of its life acquiring, preparing, enjoying, and sharing food. The taste of special favorites—*huevos rancheros* topped with salsa and fresh cilantro. A platter of pineapple, watermelon, and banana with lime squeezed over it. Creamy vanilla ice cream. No, life isn't worth it without them. Never eating is not an option. I won't stand for it. This can't be happening.

I told myself, take a deep breath, Connie. It hasn't happened yet. One thing at a time. We'll try the stent first. I'll still taste food with the stent.

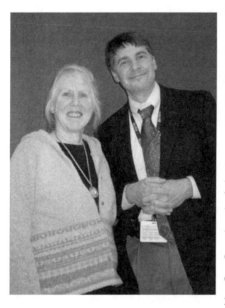

So we tried it. But, after being put to sleep to have the stent inserted, I awoke still stentless, for reasons too boring to relate.

In January of 2009, my Oregon melanoma oncologist, Dr. Brendan Curti suggested that radiation might help shrink the tumor enough to keep me eating, at least for awhile. He called the treatment "palliative," meaning it was not intended as a cure for the cancer. It was intended to treat my symptoms. The idea was to shrink the tumor enough that eating would no longer be painful. This might buy me several more months of eating on my own before the tumor started growing back. It might not work, though. Melanoma does not always respond to radiation, but we decided it was worth a try.

The first appointment at radiology was like getting fitted for a new suit. They took careful measurements and lined up the spots where the radiation would be aimed. Beams would zap me from five different directions. The five beams would intersect at the heart of the tumor. That means that each beam would do only one fifth of the damage to the surrounding healthy tissue as it would do to the center of the cancer.

To point the beams at identical angles during each radiation session they first made a customized pillow that conformed to my shape, so that each time I lay down I would be in the same position. Then they tattooed my skin with small, dark dots; three running between my breasts and two at each side of my rib cage. They're still there. Permanent reminders of my ordeal.

When the tattoo artist came at me with the needle, I asked if she would please tattoo a Virgin of Guadalupe on my chest. She said she would love to, but lacked the time.

The next morning I arrived early at the radiation facility. Following instructions from the day before, I picked out a johnny and bathrobe from a stack that had been laid out for all the radiation patients. I ushered myself into a dressing room to change. After locking my clothes in a locker, I wore the key on a wristband. Then I sat in the waiting area with other robed patients. An overhead camera surveyed the waiting area. That's how the staff knew the patient had arrived. There was no check-in. The wait was no longer than five or ten minutes before somebody called my name. There was a sci-fi surreality to this video-monitored self-check-in.

Each treatment was brief and painless. There were fifteen of them—five days a week for three weeks. Most patients receive lower doses over a longer period, but the urgency of my case called for higher doses over a short time. I would lie motionless on my custom pillow while an overhead machine whirred and blinked and moved from one side to the other. That's it. Nothing to it. I had the rest of the day to myself.

The time in the waiting room was just long enough to chat with fellow travelers and to get to know them a little, since we all had daily treatments at the same time. I met a lawyer there who recognized me from my courtroom days. He had tongue cancer, and the prognosis was good, so he wasn't too worried. I thought, what irony. A lawyer with cancer of the only part of the body a lawyer truly needs.

I met an intriguing character in the waiting room. This person had no hair, and didn't try to hide the baldness. I assumed the baldness was from chemo. This person was entirely round—round face, round body, round pudgy hands. I couldn't see whether breasts were hidden under the bathrobe, nor could I see the shape of the waist. The voice fell somewhere between male and female; deep for a woman but high for a man. Every day this person of undetermined gender was accompanied by a fellow who looked like he'd crawled out of a sleeping bag under a bridge. Although the fellow was hard-boiled and scruffy, he was kind and attentive to his companion.

Every day I greeted the two of them, and every day I looked for clues as to the gender of the person being treated. The one getting treatment was brave, loud, and cheerful. The companion was pretty much silent. I liked them. There was not a hint of self-pity in their auras.

One day I finally found out what I had wanted to know. The patient got called in before I did, and I had a chance to ask the companion, "How do you two know each other?" The fellow told me, "She's my wife."

That answers that. It still didn't answer where and how they live. They were clearly not people of means. But I got a delightful shock one day.

My radiation treatments were always early in the morning, and I liked to go to the hospital coffee shop for a fruit smoothie after I was done. The icy drink cooled my radiation-scorched throat. I was walking along the hallway, and I saw the scruffy man pushing a woman in a wheelchair. She was clearly a woman. She wore a black, long-haired, wavy wig. She wore thick make-up. Her eyes were as dark as Cleopatra's and her lips a searing red. There she was, in all her overdone glory–the man's flamboyant wife. I greeted them cheerfully and gushed about how marvelous she looked. She was delighted that I noticed.

For the first couple of weeks, I was able to drive myself to and from the treatments. I was beginning to think, piece of cake. I'll sail through this unfazed. I even went up skiing near the beginning of treatments. I got lots of praise from the staff for my stamina. I was the tough one. I was the patient who was full of piss and vinegar.

Then I wasn't. I turned marshmallow. Toward the end, I needed help. My sister and friends pitched in. They got up early without complaint to drive me to the hospital. They'd been asking what they could do for so long that I swallowed my pride and collected on those offers. Learning to ask for help has been one big lesson for an independent cuss like me. The lesson is that people want to help. Asking others for help can make them feel special and needed. I've learned that we struggling patients should not let our pride deprive our friends and family of the opportunity to be useful to us. If we up and die, we should leave them feeling they did the best they could for us. It's the polite thing to do. Think of it as cancer courtesy.

Radiation is exhausting. They literally kill a part of the body. The body goes on strike. I could hardly walk. Rather than navigate long hospital corridors on foot, I let people push me in a wheelchair. In grocery stores, I learned to drive the motorized carts they provide, so I could sit while shopping. I qualified for a handicapped parking permit. I was suddenly and severely disabled.

At home, I had stockpiled ready-to-eat food, but my throat was so burned I could barely swallow. My throat felt like scorched sandpaper, and pushing even a bite of toast past the sore spot was painful. I had zero appetite. It hurt to drink water. I forced myself to swallow fluids, but only because the doctor told me I must.

Fatigued beyond belief, I spent long hours on my couch watching movie after movie, but mostly napping and missing all the plots. One day I watched five movies in a row.

After a few days I let friends take me out to lunch, but eating was not working out for me. It not only hurt to eat, but the radiation screwed with my taste buds so I couldn't predict what I might enjoy. Since it hurt to talk, conversation was one-sided, but I treasured being out with my friends, and I was a grateful listener.

My skin got "burned" from the radiation. The front of my chest was chafed and peeling. A nurse recommended aloe vera gel. It helped heal the area rapidly without leaving the radiation scars that some people get.

I couldn't walk far, but I tried to get moving as soon as I could. A friend who came to visit accompanied me around my block. That first time it took twenty minutes to circle the block once. Several days later, I circled the block three times. I kept working my way up, but the farthest I have walked this entire year is five miles. I used to walk five miles easily every Friday morning with a hiking group. Now, one year later, it's still a big deal to walk that far.

After the radiation, I had to wait a month for my first scan, which would show whether or not the tumor had responded to the treatments. During that month I was so debilitated that I began to lose hope. I thought, what if the treatments don't work? I may never feel any better than I do right now, and right now I feel like dogshit. I thought, this could be what dying is like. You feel bad, then you feel worse, and then you're gone.

It was during that time that I banged my shin on the dishwasher door, triggering an uncontrollable crying jag. I cried, first from the pain, but the floodgates of my blocked emotions opened and I continued to cry and to mourn. For the first time, I let myself dwell on the loss that death would mean— loss to myself, and loss to those who love me. I sobbed loudly, and I followed my feelings wherever they led. They led to total despair. I could no longer dance. I could no longer ski. I wanted my life back. I yearned for everything to return to normal. The likelihood of death in the near future was real. I had no say about it. I was caught in a web of fate that generated its own timetable. I could only wait for the results of the next scan.

I gave up the struggle and turned myself over to whatever forces were battling within me. They'd have to duke it out and let me know who won. I could choose sides, but I couldn't pick the winner.

The next day after this good, long cry, and after my surrender to my fate, I felt re-energized. The full acceptance that I had no control over the outcome of my treatments was strangely liberating. I was no longer battling cancer. I was merely watching and waiting. My job was done, and I could finally relax. A weight lifted. My enthusiasm and optimism returned. I began to improve rapidly, both physically and emotionally. I took a moderate walk in the fresh air. Air tasted good. Walking felt good. Melanoma Mama was on the comeback.

Between the end of radiation and the next scan, I attended the most wonderful party. My mother celebrated her ninetieth birthday at the end of February, 2009. She had planned for the longest time to make a big deal out of her ninetieth birthday. I had dreaded for the longest time that I might die and ruin the festivities. But I didn't. Not only did I live to see Mom turn ninety, I was able to fly to Florida for the party. I traveled with my sister, Catherine, who pushed me in a wheelchair through the airport. No way could I walk those long corridors.

The party was a catered picnic under a pavilion at a Florida beach near my older sister Carol's home in a retirement community–the perfect mix of outdoor informality with elegant food. Enough people from my mother's New Hampshire town spend winters in Florida that the guests included some of Mom's close friends, as well as family. I brought a beach chair to the party, and I opened it out flat. I napped in the warm breeze under swaying palms. I thought, how strange. Here's Mom at ninety, full of pep, cheerfully greeting guests, looking for shells on the beach, sipping wine, and savoring gourmet food, and here I am, snoozing away. What's wrong with this picture? But at least I made it. I'm alive to see Mom so happy–in good health, surrounded by all four of her children, miscellaneous in-laws, a gaggle of friends and her sweet, caring husband, Frank. What a grand *fiesta*. And I didn't go and wreck it by dying.

The next scan delivered the first good medical news I had received in two years. The tumor was shrinking. Hallelujah. The radiation worked.

The next scan after that showed the tumor shrinking even more. The radiation had combined forces with the interleukin-2 in a way that the doctors hadn't expected or predicted. The radiation was supposed to be palliative only, but was doing more than planned. My own immune system had been kickstarted by the radiation/IL-2 combo.

It was during this appointment that Dr. Curti told me that

we must still be cautiously optimistic, but that I might live up to twenty more years. Drumrolls and trumpets, please. Unbelievable. What just happened? I've just been told I've got a chance to get my life back. After a year and a half of anemia. Then clobbered by major bowel surgery. Two rounds of gruesome interleukin-2. Weeks of searing radiation treatments. And now, no more treatments. Just watch the tumor shrink and stay optimistic. That was the news.

When Catherine and I walked out of the doctor's office and into the hallway, we let loose with whoops and cheers. I spun in circles, thrust my middle finger skyward and shouted, "Fuck the Grim Reaper!" We laughed 'til tears flowed.

By the time of the third scan, the tumor had gone from nine centimeters down to three. Now, one year later, the latest scan shows it even a bit smaller than that. It appears dormant.

I've gone for the better part of a year with no medical treatments whatsoever. I've flown to Florida, and to Las Vegas. I've driven twice across the country. I've climbed several mountains and I've danced and skied. I've stopped giving things away. (About the things I did give away, what am I supposed to do? Go to my friends and say, "Hey, I didn't die after all. Give me back my stuff." I don't think so.) I've bought new clothes and shoes. I even bought a bar of scented soap I didn't need. I bought a turquoise necklace in Yellowstone and a camping knife in Cody. I've played my guitar while my stepfather, Frank played flute, and boy, did we swing. I continued to study Italian, and I look forward to a trip to Italy some day. I hosted a cozy Thanksgiving dinner in the charming farmhouse kitchen.

And I wrote. I've spent months writing this book about melanoma. I wasn't going to write about it, because I thought I didn't have enough time. But time came to me in abundance–a big, silken blanket of time that delivered a luxurious, soft unfolding of light and air, and fields of sparkling snow, and hillsides of red-and-gold fall foliage, and a chilly mountain lake that seduced me to jump right in, and an endless array of food–food that I rolled over my tongue with joy and swallowed without pain–ice cream from the local creamery, and raspberries from Frank's garden, and crisp fall apples, and Maine lobster dipped in butter. Oh my, how I have eaten this year. How I have eaten.

◇◇◇◇◇

Chapter Sixteen

Of course I was delighted with my unexpected recovery. But there was one ironic downside. It was best stated by one of the women in my cancer support group who said, "When they told me I would die soon, I went out and spent all my money, and now, darn it all, it looks like I'll live."

In my case, I didn't go broke, but I was in the same boat as many retired folk who have lost value in their retirement accounts during this recession. I didn't worry about the sudden economic decline since I didn't expect to outlive my savings. But my recovery meant I was back in the business of worrying about what normal people worry about; income, and taking care of day-to-day business. For example, I had filed for an extension of the April, 2009 due date on my income taxes, and as the new October due date approached, I realized I would have to pay taxes after all. I couldn't just die and get out of it.

I'm lucky that, for me, life is more joy than burden, but with my unexpected longevity came the return of life's normal difficulties. I point this out so that others in the same boat, or the caretakers of people who get a reprieve will realize that the recovering person's feelings can be mixed, and that it is not a poke in fate's eye to sometimes lack one hundred percent gratitude.

But I digress. Back on the road, heading east across Michigan, I enjoyed a memorable, sparkling sight. In the morning light, thousands of spiderwebs glistened with dew in the grass. I didn't know whether this was a local phenomenon or whether I'd never happened to notice this unique combination of dew, morning light, and fields filled with spider webs. Either way, spiders are good. They are one of nature's insecticides, along with bats. May their webs glisten forever in the morning sun.

I saw a wild turkey crossing a field. Benjamin Franklin wanted the turkey, not the bald eagle, to be the national bird. He thought they were wily and handsome, while the eagle was only one notch more appealing than a scavenging turkey vulture. I find wild turkeys comical with their bulbous bodies, their graceless, skinny necks, and their pinheads.

Wild turkeys are everywhere now in New Hampshire. They are one of the animals that benefited from New Hampshire's reforestation. They constantly wander through the yard at the family farmhouse. Last spring, I saw a male with tail spread in full display while the nearby females studiously ignored his vanity. Later in the summer, I saw a female with her chicks strolling across the front lawn. I startled them, so Mama shooed her babies into the bushes, then flew across the street to prove to me that she was alone and childless. When I disappeared from her sight, she came back and rousted the little guys from the bushes. So I guess Mr. Fantail had his wicked way with Mama after all.

The colors on the Michigan trees are starting to turn yellow and red. It is late September, 2009 and autumn in the East begins. How lovely.

I cross the border into Canada, our misunderstood neighbor to the north. They speak English (except where they speak French) and they eat at McDonalds, so, except for their funny looking money, they're about like us. Right? Not so. Canadians on the whole take umbrage at being thought of as a northern species of U.S. citizen. They pride themselves on a broader outlook on life and a greater fondness for tea.

One noticeable difference on entering Ontario is a sense of orderliness and uniformity in the highway road signs. Whereas our unfettered free enterprise system in combination with our First Amendment right to shout louder than the next guy has fostered garish roadside billboards, in Ontario, the exit signs list gas stations, motels, and restaurants on a single sign, with each business getting the same size and style of type. Neat. Tidy. Quite British, don't you think?

Ontario farmland is flat and lush. Many rural houses are built of bricks in a decorative style distinctive to this area. I enjoy my ride through the charming countryside as I head toward London, Ontario where my cousin Ellen lives.

Ellen is an identical twin. When we were kids, I couldn't tell her apart from her sister Anne. Nobody could. Their own mother called them each "Twinny" to avoid mixing them up. Having identical, lively cousins was lots of fun. Ellen and Anne lived on a farm, which added to the fun. They taught me how to ride their palomino, Cheyenne, and how to brush him afterwards. We'd stand in the barn with its rich, horsy smell and brush Cheyenne with a wire brush that left swirls in his brown and white coat.

Anne and Ellen showed me how to stick my fingers deep into the wool of the sheep they were raising. Down inside, there's warm, oily lanolin that feels good on little fingers. They showed me how to collect eggs by reaching under the warm, plump bodies of sitting hens. You grab confidently and rapidly so you don't get pecked. They let me cuddle fuzzy yellow chicks that clustered under heat lamps for warmth.

In the 1950's I wore their hand-me-down clothes. I thought their ruffled cotton dresses were sweet, and I couldn't wait to grow into them. When they were older and were dressing for a prom, I helped them practice sitting down in Cinderella gowns that had hoop skirts underneath. They had to gently perch on the edge of the chair, because if you sink too far back with a hoop skirt on, the hoop flies up over your head, showing everything beneath. We laughed boisterously over flying hoops.

The twins were inseparable until they got married and moved apart: Anne, near Boston with her family, and Ellen to Canada with hers.

Then Anne got breast cancer. Anne struggled with cancer for years. Then she died of it. Ellen received the identical diagnosis at about the same time, but her cancer was caught in time, and was successfully treated. Ellen has never stopped mourning the loss of her twin.

As cancer survivors, Ellen and I have much to share. We sit in her sunny condominium sipping tea and Ellen tells me how cancer taught her to live in the present. She says, "For example, you've invited me for Thanksgiving, and I'm excited about coming, but I know not to project that far ahead. We're here together now, and this is the important time. Since having cancer, I've learned to appreciate what's happening around me now."

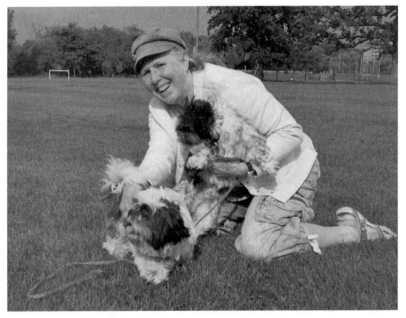

As she talks, I'm patting her two loveable rescue dogs, Lulu and Jake, brother and sister. She got them from a woman who had saved them from a puppy mill. Now Ellen lavishes these formerly neglected dogs with love and attention, and they trustingly return the favor. True to the Shih Tzu breed, they go limp in my lap like little love buckets.

Ellen also has two Maine Coon cats, Cookie and Muffin. She said that I would probably not see them, because they had been feral, and they were still exceedingly shy. Maine Coon cats are giant fluffballs, with huge padded paws that make good snowshoes. These two, mother and kitten, had been starving outdoors, and Ellen captured them and gave them a cozy place in the basement with plenty of food, but months passed before she could pat them. Her condo got remodeled without the workers ever catching sight of the elusive cats.

Ellen said, "Connie, look." Around the edge of the basement door appeared the ears and eyes of one of the cats. The cat looked at me, then ducked out of sight. Pretty soon, there it was again, its big, wild eyes staring at me. I stayed motionless on the couch.

As Ellen and I relaxed and chatted, the cat tiptoed into the room and parked itself on the rug, some distance away. It looked twice the size of a normal cat. Then it jumped onto the back of the couch near Ellen, and let Ellen pat its mound of fluff. Finally, when the cat was looking at Ellen, I sneaked my own hand onto its back and began to stroke it. It permitted me to touch it twice. I felt as proud as if I had tamed a tiger.

During my stay with Ellen, she invited her neighbor, Sue, for tea. Sue is a cheerful, rosy-cheeked woman with a hint of a Scottish accent. Sue talked enthusiastically about her plan to buy the new, one-thousand-page, hardbacked copy of the authorized biography of the Queen Mum. She says it will be interesting to read, because it goes all the way back to the scandal when King Edward the Eighth abdicated the British throne to marry the American divorcée, Mrs. Wallace Simpson. Now, for the first time, apparently, we will get the Queen Mum's take on the whole sordid affair. Oh, goody. This exemplifies another difference between Canadians and Americans. I'd sooner swallow arsenic than read a one-thousand-page authorized biography of the Queen Mum.

Another topic of discussion that highlights national differences is health care. Ellen says simply, "Here, we treat all of our sick people for free. All of them. For free." She gets upset over how American health insurance companies have manipulated public opinion to make us think that's a bad thing. She thinks the Fox News network is partly responsible for spreading the insurance companies' self-interested message.

According to Ellen, when you order a package of cable television channels in Canada, you don't automatically get the Fox News channel. They don't consider that news. They consider it right-wing propaganda. If you want Fox News, you have to specifically order the channel and pay extra.

Ellen says that the only criticism she has of their health-care system is that, unless you are seriously ill, you might have to wait a long time for an appointment. She had a glaucoma diagnosis, and it took months to see a specialist, but she says that her glaucoma was not advanced. If her condition had been critical, she would have moved to the head of the line.

I compared my own situation. With the best of America's health insurance to foot the bill, the soonest I could get my first appointment with a specialist at Dartmouth-Hitchcock was two months out. At the end of May, 2008 they scheduled my first appointment for the end of July. That was at a time when I needed blood transfusions every two weeks. A two-month delay when I was bleeding to death. Hmm. Better in Canada or the United States?

Ellen pointed out a difference in health care that makes her sad. She says that she hated to see the care her twin sister, Anne, was getting for cancer. Anne had good health insurance and was living in the Boston area where there are plenty of hospitals, but Ellen views Anne's treatment as inferior to the treatment Ellen got in Canada for the identical diagnosis.

Ellen considers moving from Canada back to the United States now that her Canadian daughter is grown and living away from home. One thing that stops her is health care. She doesn't want to switch from the Canadian system onto Medicare. She's watched her parents fight the Medicare and Medicaid bureaucracy, and she doesn't want to go through that.

Hold the presses! Fast forward to December, 2009. This story was intended to have a certain arc that would conclude with a happy ending. My cancer held in check. Connie gets a second chance after facing near certain death. That part of the story won't change. I had hoped my second chance would last maybe twenty more years. Now, I'm not sure. After close to a year's reprieve, it's back to my job as Professional Cancer Patient.

The doctors scan me every three months to watch for any recurrence of cancer. They alternate CT scans with PET scans. CT (usually pronounced "cat") stands for Computerized Tomography. PET stands for Positron Emission Tomography.

It's December of 2009, and I'm back in Oregon, home from New Hampshire after my cross-country camping trip and after several peaceful autumn months in the New Hampshire family farmhouse writing this book. In mid-December I had a PET scan at Providence Hospital in Portland. They injected me with radioactive gunk and I drank a "contrast" of who-knows-what. I lay on a bed that slid back and forth through a big, white doughnut, which took pictures of my innards, head to toe. Anyplace where the radioactive goop concentrates will show up in the pictures. It has to do with cancer being a glutton for glucose, which shows up as hot spots. My last scan, six months ago, showed nothing new; only the Incredible Shrinking Tumor in my chest.

This latest scan was in mid-December. Here's my Christmas present. A new lump spotted. That's not how I planned this story. The book was supposed to start and finish with my cross-country camping trip, Oregon to New Hampshire, during which I would be remembering the trials and tribulations of my treatments the year before. I hadn't planned to include the long drive home from New Hampshire to Oregon, since I scurried home with little sightseeing during the cold of December. But that trip in itself turned into another adventure. Here's the Reader's Digest version that I sent to friends and family:

December 15, 2009: For those who wonder how my cross-country drive was, I'm now safely home in Oregon after many adventures of the bad-weather and broken-down-car variety. But the grueling ordeal was worth it. I got to ski in the Colorado Rockies. (Never mind that it was nine below and at an oxygen-poor 10,000 feet. I had fun.) I also got to view the majestic, snow-covered Tetons from a remote Wyoming road, as if they were presenting themselves to me alone—my personal wintery Christmas card. I also got to stay in places like "The Stagecoach Inn", and "The Buffalo Lodge", and eat in places like "The Cowboy Cafe." To top it all off, I got stranded by weather in a remote town called Chugwater, Wyoming, home of the famous "Chugwater Chili Cook-Off."

So, after weather delays and one day of sitting in a car repair shop, I made it home to Oregon on a Sunday afternoon in mid-December, 2009, just in time to go in for my scheduled PET scan on Monday morning. I was in good spirits because I had been feeling well in my chest area, and I was expecting excellent results.

I find PET scans relaxing, because I'm lying still, the machine is quiet, and I can see the room around me. While the bed moves back and forth through the doughnut hole, I meditate. When I meditate, I envision a bright spot in the center of my forehead, and I mentally repeat a simple mantra to keep my mind from wandering. I breathe slowly and evenly. By the time the scan was finished, I was relaxed and refreshed.

The day after my scan, I went to see my West Coast melanoma oncologist, Dr. Brendan Curti. He's a cute little bugger, but unfortunately he's a Yankees fan, which doesn't sit well with Red Sox supporters. I have to put him and my Sox-fan sister Catherine in separate corners.

In spite of my doctor's baseball-induced blind spot, he's a brilliant guy who takes all the time needed to explain things. He came into the room, limping. One leg was bound in a plastic brace from a squash injury. He asked me how I was doing. "Better than you, apparently," I said.

He gave me the good and bad news. The good news was that the Incredible Shrinking Tumor had shrunk a bit more. I asked about its chances of growing back. He said, "Only two in ten." That means there's an eighty percent chance that I'm done with that sucker. It's not life-threatening now, and may never be so again.

Now for the bad news. The scan showed a one-inch diameter spot in my left buttock. I looked at the picture and could see the spot, in the tissue, not too far in. It was not engaged with any major organs, so it was removable.

Now for the silver lining. Remember how they wanted to make a vaccine from my abdominal tumor but couldn't? This lesion looks good for "harvesting" for a personal vaccine.

Vaccines are not yet standard treatment. If they can make a vaccine from this rotten spot, I will participate in a clinical trial—a scientific study on the effectiveness of the vaccine. I won't go into detail now because I have yet to qualify for any clinical trial. Something always rules me out. Let's wait and see.

Tomorrow is Christmas Eve, 2009. Mom and Frank fly in tonight from New Hampshire. Thanks to the scheduling gods, my surgery got squeezed in before Christmas and I'm recovering just fine.

Yesterday morning at 5:30 a.m., my neighbor Chris drove me to the hospital. Chris is the same neighbor who helped me load up my camping gear last September and who snowshoed with me into downtown Portland. On the way to the hospital, I thanked him for getting up so early, and he burst into song: "You're not heavy. You're my neighbor."

My sister Catherine, who is normally my West Coast support person, couldn't accompany me to the hospital because she and her family were in a flurry of activity moving into a lovely new home, racing to unpack enough boxes that they can entertain us all at Christmas.

My surgery began with a CT scan during which the technicians inserted a wire into the tumor so that the surgeon could follow the wire to find his way to the exact spot. I saw on the scan that they nailed that puppy dead center with the wire. Good work.

Then they gave me la la juice through my IV so I'd stay calm while being rolled into the operating room, where they dripped in the beddy-bye cocktail. Lights out.

When I awoke, it was not my butt that was sore, but my

throat. They jab in a breathing tube during the operation that turns your throat into a Pennsylvania highway (some of the roughest roads in the nation). I thrashed, fighting not to wake up to the pain, so they slipped some morphine in my IV, and I happily extended my nap. When I next awoke, I could face the world. In fact, I snapped out of it quickly and was able to walk on my own.

Here's an email I sent to friends and family:

December 22, 2009: A quick update. Surgery today went well—no hitches. La la juice is still making me loopy. Feeling no pain. I'm home and moving around, fixing my own food, and sitting on a doughnut pillow to protect the area that now features Frankenstein stitches across my formerly sexy bottom. Bye bye bikini. (Oops, forgot. I kissed that bikini goodbye long ago.) The rotten spot has been carved out of there, but I don't know yet the details about turning it into a vaccine. More on this later. For now, it's a high and happy Christmas for this kid.

You can see I maintain a pretty bright outlook most of the time. How did I really feel when I got this new diagnosis? Like crap. I've been thrilled at the idea that my own immune system has been finding the cancer. It struck me hard to learn that another spot was growing in me. I've been going through the motions of getting ready for Christmas, without much yuletide spirit. But last year at this time, I didn't even put up a tree or decorations, so I'm ahead of the game this year. But I'm tired of wondering whether I'll live to see another Christmas. That movie gets old.

Two years ago, it was the anemia that dragged me down at Christmas. At the winter solstice I danced at a "blindfolded trance dance." Dancing blindfolded brings you inward to connect with whatever's going on. At that time I knew only that I was battling anemia of undiagnosed cause. I remember that, during the dance, I was lying on the floor with my hand on the very spot on my belly from which a tumor was later surgically removed. I was kneading that sore spot and crying inconsolably. I know now that while I danced that night, my body told my brain that I was in serious trouble. Thus the copious tears. Without realizing that I had a cancerous tumor, I was mourning my upcoming demise.

Last year, I was crawling out of the hole of interleukin-2 treatments and heading toward the wonderful world of radiation. I lacked the festive spirit and didn't host my annual holiday dinner.

This year, I have planned a Christmas feast and have decorated my home in my own style. My Mexican folk-art masks are now wearing Santa hats and reindeer antlers, and my pagan goddess statue is strewn with festive strands of colored ornaments. My closest friends will come, and they'll get to see Mom and Frank, and we'll enjoy warmth and cheer and love. I don't know if this will be my last Christmas.

When I imply my days might be numbered, people sometimes say, "None of us know how long we'll live." As if we're all in the same boat. As if I'm supposed to agree that it doesn't matter to me that I've been diagnosed with an incurable, life-threatening disease, because, after all, life is sure to end for all of us. Sorry, but I can't be so sanguine about it. I'm not saying this to garner the sympathy vote, but having Stage IV melanoma is not the same as knowing, generally, that all living things must die. It just isn't. Knowing that I can theoretically get crunched by a speeding train or knocked on the bean by a meteorite is not the same as the day-to-day realization that there's an enemy lurking in me that loves to suck my blood and grow out of control in all kinds of inconvenient places. I don't like it. I hate it.

It's not about fairness—I don't often spend time moaning, "Why me?"

It's not about not having lived yet. If there's some pleasure, licit or illicit that I've missed out on in life, I honestly can't think of it. I'm a fiend for sucking up life, rare and juicy.

It's not about not having contributed enough good yet. Of course I could do more, but I'm proud of my accomplishments.

Here's what it's about. Being sick just plain sucks. It's like being trapped on a nausea-producing carnival ride that won't stop to let you off. It's about feeling helpless in a cruel, cold universe that wantonly wipes out whole species, and doesn't give a flying fuck about one struggling human.

My melanoma has proved that it can pop up at any place at any time. This time I got lucky. In many other spots it would not be so easily removable. If it passes the blood-brain barrier, it can move into the important wiring that makes me who I am. If it passes into the liver, pancreas, or lungs, watch out. I'm not liking this at all. Maybe they can make the vaccine. I'll update you when I know. Maybe a vaccine will work. Maybe it won't. But I'm the Melanoma Mama, and I'm still taking names and still kicking ass. Don't mess with the Melanoma Mama!

◇◇◇◇◇

Chapter Seventeen

After leaving cousin Ellen's London, Ontario home, I crossed back into the United States at Niagara Falls. I like Niagara Falls. It's big. It's tacky. It makes me wish I'd married a New Jersey plumber, so we could have honeymooned there.

I doubt many people go to Niagara Falls for honeymoons anymore like they did in the old movies. Back then, all people could afford was a not-too-lengthy ride in the car and one night in a cheap motel. Now, many people fly to tropical resorts for their honeymoons. They even have "destination" weddings in remote locales. They force their guests to cough up airfare, meals, and lodging on top of a suitably expensive wedding gift. The chutzpah of some people.

When we took our family trip to Yellowstone back in 1959, we stopped at Niagara Falls. We put on rain ponchos and rode on the Maid of the Mist. I remember the excitement of riding the boat in close where the falls roared and soaked us while we imagined crashing over the falls, with or without a barrel, and splattering our guts on the rocks. Kids love to imagine nifty ways to die.

This time, I watched as the boats, each called Maid of the Mist, plied their way into the spray that rose and churned at the foot of the falls. The boats were loaded with tourists in blue slickers. I was tempted to take a ride for old time's sake, but frankly, it was cold, and the mist that reached me where I stood at the viewpoint chilled me. Instead, I enjoyed watching the multi-national parade of tourists taking each other's photos in front of the giant falls.

I tried to picture what it would have been like to come across these falls hundreds of years ago, while out in the wilderness, but the city setting is so integral to them now that Niagara Falls without casinos, and without tourist traps like Ripley's Believe It or Not, and without impossible traffic, just wouldn't be the same. And in this regard, Canada is an even worse offender than the United States, probably because its better view of the falls has drawn more greed and bad taste.

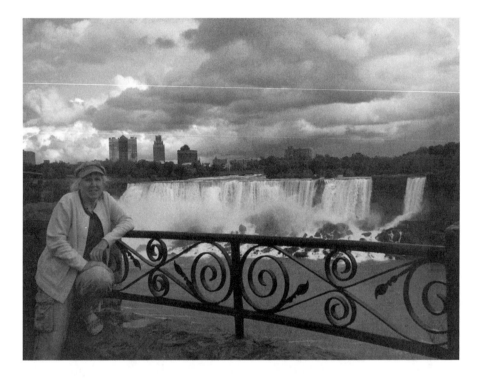

I once read a description that Margaret Fuller wrote of Niagara Falls. Margaret Fuller was a writer and an intellectual who liked to hang out with Uncle Ralph. She tried to convince him to let her edit his writing, but he believed in the immediacy of the first draft, and wasn't going to let either her or Henry David Thoreau tinker with his words. I too believe in the immediacy of the first draft. First thought, best thought. But

Ralph Waldo Emerson could have used a good editor. He was a riveting public speaker, tall for the era, with piercing eyes that mesmerized an audience. But his writing, for all its flashes of brilliance, is a bit opaque. Sorry, Uncle Ralph, but it's true.

Anyway, in 1843, Margaret Fuller wrote about her impressions of the falls in her book, *Summer on the Lakes*. With typical nineteenth century hyperbole, she waxed poetic about how the surging waters stir the breast and whatnot, but her true feelings show through, and mirror my own. She wrote, "For the magnificence ... of the falls I was prepared by descriptions and by paintings. When I arrived in sight of them, I merely felt, 'ah, yes, here is the fall, just as I have seen it in picture.'"

The area around the falls was already getting built up back in 1843. Margaret Fuller writes, "People complain of the buildings at Niagara, and fear to see it further deformed. I cannot sympathize with such an apprehension: the spectacle is capable to swallow up all such objects; they are not seen in the great whole, more than an earthworm in a wide field." I guess there were no multi-story casinos back then.

She imagined, as I did, what the falls were like before the encroachment of civilization. She says, "The perpetual trampling of the waters seized my senses ... Continually upon my mind came, unsought and unwelcome, images, such as never haunted it before, of naked savages stealing behind me with uplifted tomahawks; again and again this illusion recurred, and even after I had thought it over, and tried to shake it off, I could not help starting and looking behind me." I, myself, imagined bears and raccoons feeding at the riverside, but being attacked by naked savages never once crossed my mind. Hers was a different era.

After leaving the falls, I went north to the New York shore of Lake Ontario. I chose that northern route to get off the interstate highway. It was a good choice. The route included many views of the lake, plus orchards with deep red apples ripening on the trees—so many apples, the trees looked more red than green.

I was happy to be pitching my tent again, even though the weather was cool and the campground at Hamlen Beach State Park was nearly deserted. From the array of abandoned sites, I chose a site near enough to other campers that they could hear my battery-powered siren or my yelling if needed, but not so near that they would notice I was a woman camping alone in a largely uninhabited place.

When I checked into the campground, I saw a photo on the wall of New York's governor, David Paterson. I remembered that he had replaced the former governor, Eliot Spitzer when Spitzer got caught with his pants down. Now Spitzer is trying to reinvent himself as a television talk show pundit.

Usually I ignore sex scandals. It never surprises me when guys in power get caught womanizing. I've read too much about alpha chimps in the wild. The evolutionary reason the male primate risks life and limb to become head honcho is because that gives him access to the choice females. So, when the human version of the alpha chimp gets to the top of the heap, what's he do? He goes for the hot babes. It's basic biology.

In Spitzer's case, I admit to becoming intrigued by the drama of his downfall. Spitzer had been excessively self-righteous in his crusades against white-collar criminals when he was New York's attorney general. Not that many of his targets didn't deserve it, but there was a stench of egomania behind Spitzer's high-profile prosecutions. He's the kind of guy we love to see topple from grace. And it was his own stupid fault, because he was such a classic trick.

Spitzer paid thousands of dollars every time he wanted to get laid. It cost so much, he had to funnel the money through secret accounts. That's how he got caught. For a supposedly smart guy, that's stupid. He never figured out that pussy is pussy and one orgasm is as good as the next. He had to do it in style. Did he really get more bang for his buck than the guy who pays twenty dollars for a back seat blow job? All Spitzer got was a nicer hotel room and a girl who smiled at him. Beyond that, a hooker's a hooker.

I figured out that orgasms know no class distinctions when I represented an incarcerated client, a Mexican farmworker, who wanted me to retrieve personal items out of his crashed car. I found a notebook with somebody's cartoonish sketches of people having fun with their oversized genitalia. It was the poor man's homemade porn. I realized that sex can be enjoyed equally by the poor and the rich. In fact, I bet that my farmworker client enjoyed sex more than Spitzer because my client wasn't an uptight jerk.

I settled in happily at the lakeside campground, and that night I had the most marvelous dream. I dreamt that I had discovered the most beautiful campground in the world, and that it was here, on Lake Ontario. I dreamt that when I got up in the morning, the sun shined as warmly as in mid-summer, and skies were clear and blue. I wore a frothy, white dress that floated over my body, rippling in the breeze, like in a shampoo commercial. The lake danced with gentle waves that licked the pure-white, sandy shore. I walked barefoot on the beach and felt warm, fine sand caress my feet. In my dream, I was delirious with joy.

There may be days when this campground matches my lovely dream, but the next morning was not one of them. I awoke to the drizzle of rain on my tent. The drizzle escalated to a roaring downpour. It was still dark out, but I hurried to pack up my gear. I had to plan carefully to keep from getting soaked. I got dressed while hunched in my bubble of a tent. I knelt on the hard tent floor while packing my nighty, book, flashlight, and such into my overnight bag. I stayed hunched in the dry tent while stuffing my sleeping bag in its duffel bag and sucking the air out of the mattress with a battery-operated pump. Once I had everything, including my red Folger's pee pot, in neat piles, I donned my rain poncho and dashed for the car with my gear. I disassembled my tent in record time, and threw it in a soaking heap on top of everything. I didn't try to fix breakfast, but planned to stop for a warm, dry meal along the highway. So much for skipping along Lake Ontario's sunshiny shore.

I was in for another long day of highway driving in the pouring rain. Anxious to get home to family and friends, I resigned myself to a boring drive along the rain-soaked New York Thruway in competition with the big beasts whose tires continuously flung water at me.

As I drive, I calculate that I'm only one day away from Dartmouth-Hitchcock Hospital where cousin Steve is recovering from surgery for his rectal cancer. I'll soon be returning to the torture chambers where I suffered my own abdominal surgery the year before, and where I endured my two sessions in the pits of interleukin's hell.

In New York, close to three thousand miles from my Oregon home, I'm feeling fine. Great, in fact. I'm proud that I'm capable of all this travel. Here it is, late September, and only the prior February I was struggling to travel from my couch to the kitchen for a glass of water. That winter of 2009 I had told my cancer support group that I could picture the upcoming summer, but when it came to the fall, a grey curtain dropped over my imagination. My mental calendar turned summer's sunny corner and dissolved into darkness. I felt, not so much fearful, as adrift with uncertainty.

Now the fall that I couldn't picture is clearly in focus with its orange-tinged leaves, its ripening apples, and even its pouring rain. I'm here. I'm alive. I'll happily take whatever this fall dishes out.

After a long day of tedious thruway driving in the rain, by late afternoon I made it across the New York border into Bennington, Vermont. Bennington is the town where the poet Robert Frost is buried. The bittersweet epitaph on his gravestone reads, "I had a lover's quarrel with the world."

Bennington also boasts the Bennington Museum, which houses a large collection of paintings by the famous primitive painter, Grandma Moses, who began painting at age seventy-six. She had advancing arthritis and could no longer embroider, but she found she could hold a paintbrush. She continued to paint until her death in 1961 at age 101, and by that time she had produced more than 1,000 paintings and had become world famous. She was born before Lincoln was elected president, and she liked to paint what she called "old-timey" pictures to show people how things used to be.

I had driven through Bennington on other occasions, but the timing was never right to stop and tour the museum. I had always wanted to see it. This time, after driving across New York since before sunrise, I was ready for a break. I planned to view the art, and I was resting on a bench inside the museum, getting ready to purchase my admission ticket when I thought I'd better first call my Uncle Bill and let him know my plans, which were to tour the museum, stop early for a good night's rest, then pick him up in the morning to take him to the hospital to see Steve.

"Hey, Uncle Bill. I'm in Bennington, Vermont. Getting closer." I told him my plans.

"Stay overnight?" he said. "I thought you were coming today. I'd hoped to see Steve tonight."

"I'm so tired. It's been a long drive."

"It's only a couple more hours to Hanover."

A couple more hours. Ouch. "All right, Uncle Bill. I'm coming."

My cousin's surgery had been days ago and his father was anxious to see him. Uncle Bill's advanced diabetes had gone to his legs, and he could no longer drive. If anybody knows the importance of having family support during recovery from surgery, it's me. Grandma Moses' paintings will be there on my next trip through. I pushed on.

Vermont is legendary for its romantic, rural character. Even though it was still raining, the road from Killington to White River Junction was lovely. It wound along beside a rocky river framed with yellowing fall foliage.

Going by the ski area at Killington reminded me of the last time I had gone skiing with Uncle Bill. One of his knees would no longer support him, but he loved to ski. He favored his bum knee by making wide, arcing turns on his good side. Then he stopped to step around when his bad knee wouldn't take the pressure of the next turn. But he enjoyed being out there doing what he could. That's where I get it from. His generation, including my father, my mother, and my Uncle Art (who was known as Ski Wax in New Hampshire's White Mountains in the 1930's) all skied until it was impossible to continue. They taught me to enjoy what you can while you can. Just keep at it.

Uncle Bill also taught me how to laugh about death. One crisp fall day in 1994, the family stood in solemn ceremony beside a gravestone in an old New England cemetery while a cool breeze rustled the maple leaves, and the sun shone in a clear blue sky. My father's ashes lay inside a golden box that sat beside the gravestone, ready for burial. Uncle Bill, who had metal knee replacements, looked at the box containing the ashes of his brother, and I overheard him whisper to his wife Midge, "I don't think you'll get me in that box. My knees won't fit." Auntie Midge whispered back, "Don't worry, dear. I'm keeping them for door knockers."

As it turns out, Uncle Bill outlived his childhood sweetheart, Midge. He lives independently in an apartment at a retirement community in Hanover, New Hampshire, near Dartmouth College. I arrived at his place dog-tired, but somehow rallied the energy needed to take him to see his son Steve in the hospital.

Getting Uncle Bill in and out of his wheelchair and in and out of the car was a bit tricky, because his bum leg wouldn't bend enough to stuff his foot into the car. I was so tired and giddy that the struggle struck me funny and I started laughing. Luckily, so did he.

Dartmouth-Hitchcock Hospital is a sprawling array of medical buildings surrounded by various parking lots, but Uncle Bill knew exactly which parking lot was nearest to Steve's room. It's not a good thing to know a hospital inside-out like my family knows this place. And for me, there was the added dimension of *déjà vu*. The soft tone of elevator bells, the staff bustling silently in scrubs, carrying clipboards, the odor of cleaning products barely masking a more sinister smell, and the unreal glow cast on everything from the overhead florescent lighting all brought me back to the year before when I was the patient.

I wheeled Uncle Bill into Steve's room, and we were not pleased with what we saw. Steve was approaching the day that they originally said he might go home after his colon surgery, and he was in no shape to go anywhere. He lay back in his reclining chair, a tube in his nose and tubes in his arm. He wore an all-too-familiar, light green johnny. He was covered with one of their flimsy, cotton blankets, too thin to keep a gnat warm. He knew us, and could communicate some, but he was exhausted. Mentally, he faded in and out.

My first impression was strong. That was me. That was me last year. I wore that same johnny and reclined in that same chair and was hooked up to the same tubes. And I was that disoriented. Oh, what I must have put my mother through!

Steve's problem mirrored mine. After his surgery, his bowels wouldn't wake up. He was bloated and uncomfortable and unable to eat or drink. In his case, his nausea prompted them to shove a tube through his nose and down his throat to empty the bile from his stomach, so he wouldn't vomit. He cursed the incompetent bumbler who almost choked him to death in the process. No way would Steve let the same guy try again. He insisted on a different person. Good for you, Steve. You've got to stand up for yourself.

I'm the same way with technicians who can't find a vein when they stick a needle in my arm. I used to give them three chances to stick me, but after too many black and blue marks from too many blown veins, I'm down to one try before I holler for a supervisor.

The color of the stuff that came up Stephen's tube from his stomach was a sickening yellow. I flashed to a time I had seen a similar tube coming out of my mother. Her stomach contents had been green. Who knew that stomach juice comes in different colors, none pleasant to view.

Stephen's phone rang. It was his business partner. Steve drowsily told him to call back in the morning. He couldn't focus to talk. Boy, do I remember that problem.

Steve drifted in and out of awareness. Uncle Bill looked at me and shook his head. I said, "Maybe it's the medication. Maybe he has his ups and downs, and we just came when he's down. That's what happened to me."

I went to use the bathroom. More *déjà vu*. There's some

chemical–perhaps a cleaning product–a chemical odor that only exists in the bathrooms at Dartmouth-Hitchcock. My stomach suddenly churned and I came near to vomiting. Odors are such strong transporters across time. Of all our senses, the sense of smell can most vividly recreate a past experience with just one whiff. My whiff of that chemical transported me back to the bathroom following surgery, when that smell blended with the putrid smell of my own, suddenly unleashed bowels. I also flashed back to the bathroom of the interleukin room and tasted my bitter vomit. The vivid flashbacks were intolerable and unavoidable. I felt dizzy and sick. My only consolation was realizing that I was not the patient this time. Get a grip, Connie. You don't have to stay. This time, you can walk out the hospital door.

On the way out, Uncle Bill told me that this was the worst Stephen had been since the surgery. I sensed he feared his son was slipping away. I could only assure him that I had recovered from the identical problem.

I spent the night at Steve's home, and in the morning it was his wife Laarni's turn to visit him. I was again the taxi driver. But first, we enjoyed a leisurely bacon and egg breakfast, and I got to know her better. I'm a pushover for any heart-rending, coming-to-America immigrant story, and Laarni's was a good one.

In the Philippines, she was a young, single mother struggling to make her way. Stephen, an architect, was working over there. He met her at work, but she left her job to start nursing school, so he went looking for her. He tracked her down, but she paid little attention. He was fit and good-looking, but much older than she, and she was in no mood for someone who wasn't serious. Stephen proved steadfast over several months. He finally asked her parents for her hand, and the deal was sealed.

She left everything and everybody she knows to marry the man she loves. And now that he's sick and worried over finances, and worried about raising her daughter, Johnnice and their new baby, little Midgie, she tells him, "I've been poor all my life. I don't care about money. I care about you. Just get well."

That morning at the hospital, Steve was alert and feeling better. I was right about him having ups and downs. He greeted Laarni with hugs and kisses, and cradled his baby. He and I, having gone through similar surgeries, shared hospital stories like a couple of wounded veterans. We shared the brotherhood of the IV, the scarred belly, and the unmoved bowel. Then the phone rang, and it was the business partner with whom he'd been unable to speak the night before. It seemed important, so I suggested to Laarni that we go down to the oncology wing, because I wanted her to take my picture there, under the sign to my doctor's office.

I had Laarni snap photos of me standing, strong and proud in front of the Norris Cotton Cancer Center sign where I had spent so much time the year prior. Then in the waiting area, I had her snap more pictures by the doorway that led to Dr. Ernstoff's office. The sign overhead says, "Hematology Oncology." For the photos, I was swaggering. I posed with the confidence of an athlete who's just won the marathon. I drew in a lungful of air, because I could. I stood straight and tall and practically yipped for joy. I even blurted out to strangers in the waiting room, "I wasn't supposed to be here by now, and look at me. I'm a success story. I made it."

My joy was infectious. People's faces brightened. I hope I didn't hurt the feelings of those in the waiting room who wouldn't get a second chance, but I doubt it. I know from my cancer support group that we cancer patients are like a team— we root for the high scorer even if it doesn't happen to be us.

We're sponges soaking up hope.

Anything to offset the stark reality we face. Coping with cancer. There are many strategies, but all patients find something that helps—something to keep us from feeling trapped in the heart of darkness—something that holds back the horror. Look around this waiting room. Some of these people will die soon. There are the elderly in wheelchairs. There are young men—physically fit workers who will get beaten down by this beast. There are well-dressed women who wear lipstick and pearl necklaces to their doctors' appointments. Their manicures are perfect, but they cover their heads with scarves to hide the baldness from chemotherapy. They're here now, but in weeks, months, less than a year, some of them will be dead. But nobody is crying or cursing God. They are reading magazines, chatting with a relative, staring at the clock, and rechecking their watches. Most patients simply put one foot in front of the other. We focus on the medical procedure at hand. We pay attention only to the next blood draw, the next scan, the next radiation treatment. We don't dwell on what comes after.

It occurred to me that Dr. Ernstoff might be here today. I would like to see him again. But of course I don't have an appointment. Oh, heck. Why not give it a try?

On a whim, I went up to the receptionist. I said, "I'm one of Doctor Ernstoff's success stories. I'm writing a book called *Melanoma Mama*. I was wondering if he happens to be here today and if he'd be willing to come out and have his picture taken."

The receptionist was happy to check for me. I doubt she'd heard this one before. Within only a few minutes the receptionist said, "He'll see you."

How about that? I had to wait two months for my first appointment with a doctor in this place, but now, either the doctor wanted to see the smiling results of his good medical work, or he wanted to be sure to get his photo in the book. In either case, he came right out.

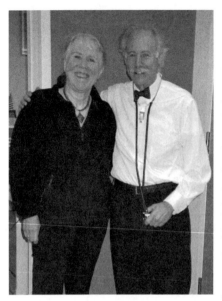

The smiling doctor, with his Groucho Marx mustache, his tousled hair, and his goofy bow tie was delighted to see me looking so happy and healthy. It must be terrible being a melanoma oncologist. The majority of your patients will die sooner or later, no matter how hard you work or how much you care. Success stories are few and far between.

He posed for photos, one with him standing alone, and one of him with his arm around his star patient. He told me he had been following my case. Dr. Curti sends him copies of the medical reports from Oregon. He was as happy as Dr. Curti that the tumor keeps shrinking. He agreed that the combination of the IL-2 working with the radiation did the trick. He confirmed that the radiation reduces the number of regulatory T-cells, which leaves the melanoma cells with no place to hide from the immune system, which has been massively boosted by the IL-2. He was glad that, after our initial disappointment, that all my suffering through IL-2 had benefited me after all.

We hugged and said goodbye. I left there glowing with happiness. I thought, good. Now I have a happy ending for my book.

Laarni and little Midgie and I went to say goodbye to Steve who, at this writing, is doing well with no recurrence of his cancer. And Uncle Bill is still hanging in there.

I only had a couple of hours of driving left on my cross-country adventure. I crossed New Hampshire, past mountains I have climbed, past lakes in which I have enjoyed swimming, to arrive in mid-afternoon in my cherished little village. I have never named the town in this book, nor will I. I learned my lesson from the time a national magazine published a list of the "best swimming holes in America," and the list included our favorite pristine river. It soon went from one of the best swimming holes in America to one of the most crowded swimming holes in America, just from that brief mention in the national press. I won't make that mistake here. There are plenty of lovely New Hampshire villages. If you want to try one out, take your pick.

I arrived in the town adjacent to ours, and I took a turn onto the road that would lead the last eight miles past an unspoiled lake with a view of a mountain range on its far side. Our family tradition is that, when we have been away, we guess the number of cars we will meet on this stretch of road. We have been coming here since I was born, and the number is pretty much constant. It is almost always somewhere between zero and ten to twelve cars, most often, fewer than five. With so little traffic you can see why I'm keeping mum about the town's name.

The center of town is always a welcome sight for weary eyes. It is a Grandma Moses painting, a Currier and Ives etching, a Norman Rockwell kind of town with white buildings dating back two hundred years. Its classic churches are worthy of an appearance on any sparkling Christmas card. I drove past the center of town and turned off onto the dirt road where Mom and Frank live. I thought I'd drop in on them before settling into the farmhouse.

I drove up their road on the last day of September, 2009 when the trees were working their way toward the peak of their fall colors. I saw a couple out walking their dog down the dirt road. It was no surprise to me that in this small town, I knew them. Tom and Mary. Tom had once driven me to Dartmouth-Hitchcock as one of the Caregivers—volunteers who help people get to medical appointments. Mary is a go-getter member of the Over the Hill Hikers club, which my mother helped found more than thirty years ago. I stopped in the middle of the road and we chatted. This happens all the time on these back roads. I have often come up behind a stopped car, and I would never think to honk and interrupt the friendly chit-chat that is taking place in the middle of the road. In this town, we politely wait for the conversation to end.

Mary and Tom reminded me that it was Mom and Frank's bridge day. They had just walked by the house and had seen them inside playing bridge with the two Jims, also Over the Hill Hikers. I said, "I guess they won't want to see me then. I'll just let them know I've arrived, and I'll come back later."

Sure enough, after all my adventures, I arrived to barely a "Hello, Connie" before their conversation turned back to, "Two no trump." It didn't hurt my feelings one bit. I am so glad that Mom and Frank have things in their lives they are so passionate about that everything else takes a back seat. Wednesday bridge day is sacred. I said hello and goodbye, and I went on home to the farmhouse.

I drove back down the dirt road and paused as I went past Tom and Mary, still out walking. "You were right," I said. "They didn't even want to see me." We all laughed. They know about Mom and Frank and bridge day.

On Friday morning, my alarm clock woke me. I get up early on Mondays, Wednesdays and Fridays to go to Colleen's exercise class in the town hall. She has been running her exercise class for so long that I'm the second generation in my family to go there. Mom and Dad used to be regulars. Dad has been dead for fifteen years, and Mom and Frank now exercise at home, three mornings a week, seated in chairs, lifting their hand weights.

I arrived at the town hall where Dad used to sing tenor in the Gilbert and Sullivan operettas that the local theater group produced each summer during my childhood. I greeted my friends. There was Ann, the other Melanoma Mama, all chipper and well. There was Dick, the haphazard gardener who had grown the runaway pumpkins that had spread all over his driveway. There were Mary and Dale and Robin and Bob and Jeff and all the rest of them, dedicated to fitness and to Colleen, who earns a bit extra by leading this class, but who would probably do it anyway, because her calling is to keep the older crowd healthy and happy.

On the way into the building I had greeted the goose and the two ducks. Behind the town hall, in the pond—a mirror that reflects the Methodist church and the gold and red maple trees— the three waterfowl hang out every day. I quack and honk my greetings. Everybody knows them, and they know everybody. Think I'm exaggerating? We have a town bulletin board on the Internet, and here are two recent messages about the goose and the two ducks:

Question: A couple of people have asked if the goose on the town hall pond could be the one we are missing. Does anyone know where that one came from or who he belongs to? I would be surprised if ours got that far from here, but we want to go get him if he's ours.

Answer: The goose at the Town Hall Pond is Beverly. She was one of Josh's geese, but after she lost her third mate to the wild things, we gave her to the Browns because they have ducks. So she and the ducks winter at the Brown's house and summer at the Town Pond. Beverly knows her name and likes to talk to people, so do stop and say hi to her. I do all the time and she does remember Cindy and me when she hears us. Al

I've lived a long and adventurous life. I've rocked out with the hippies in Golden Gate Park. I've been locked in jail cells interviewing murderers and rapists. I've watched Mount St. Helens blow its top. I've soared down snow-packed slopes with wild abandon. In all that time, I've learned only one thing. My joy is wherever I find it. My joy is usually right in front of my nose. The simple pleasure of quacking my hellos to Beverly and her two pals was my joy that morning. A person needs nothing more in life.

I don't know how much longer I'll live. I've made it past my original expiration date, and I'm thrilled every day just to be here. I'm waiting for word on whether the vaccine can be made from the tumor they just removed. I don't know what the treatments will be like or whether they will help. I only know that food tastes delicious and the touch of a human hand is a delight.

I've learned much from the wonderful women in my cancer support group. The group is called, appropriately, *Making Today Count.* We have all been diagnosed with late-stage cancer. There are other support groups for the novices, but we call ourselves the "scary" group. We get down, and we get real. When one of us dies, we have a brief ceremony called "passing the candle." Our unofficial photographer, Kathrine, passes a photo of the woman from her bulging photo album. We each say a few words.

We are told by our group facilitators that stress relief in any form is good for us—it has been shown to boost the immune system. They don't claim our cancer will be cured solely by alternative means, but we learn to contribute to our own well-being. We meditate. We listen to quiet voices that urge us to imagine ourselves in a quiet meadow by a stream—to imagine our selves strong and well. We share handouts on healthy diets, on the grieving process, on the role of caregivers, on the role of hospice. We are encouraged to dive into art, into exercise, into whatever gives us joy. We learn to plan our goodbyes—to make photo albums for those we'll leave behind. Mostly we laugh. That is, whenever we are not crying.

One time we discussed our purpose in life. When you're young and healthy, you can dream big dreams. Change the world. Make a big splash. What about now? I remember one woman saying that enjoying each day was enough now. She had realized that this is not selfish. Everybody knows she's dying. Yet they see her mostly happy. She is not keeping a stiff upper lip for the sake of appearances. She is mostly being truly happy. That gives other people hope—when they see us with our terminal diagnoses, laughing and loving and living. That's our new job. That's our purpose. To show the world how much living there is in dying. We bear the torch of hope.

I've learned to accept my state of medical limbo with all its ups and downs. I've learned to speak gently to my melanoma. It is, after all, just a warped version of myself. Here's an example of one of my recent conversations with my melanoma:

Let light and air into the body. Let it find the melanoma. Let it move the melanoma. Let it nudge it loose, scattering its debris into the blood, washing it away like sin on a tide of life—a tide of ebbing, flowing energy that does not feed its greedy lust, but surrounds it and pushes and prods it.

The melanoma says, I guess I'll go. I'll tiptoe on out. Sorry to bother you. I didn't know I was killing you. I was just doing what melanoma does.

And I say, I won't scream at you, because you might thrive on anger's juice. But I tell you, move along. There's nothing for you here. I don't need you, even though I am the Melanoma Mama. I'll gladly give up my title if you'll hit the road. Swing low, sweet melanoma. Please don't carry me home. Move, slide, ease on out. Goodbye.

◇◇◇◇◇

Chapter Eighteen

This book is now ending. I've had my say on lots of things—on the joys of cross-country camping, on the speed of light, on the Lewis and Clark expedition, and on the ethical way to slaughter a goat. You know what my surgical scars look like—the River Nile on my tummy and a Frankenstein scar on my butt. You know what interleukin-2 treatments feel like, complete with vomiting and diarrhea. I've tried to be brutally honest about death, and about hope and despair, but I've tried to focus mostly on how I have lived intensely so as not to miss what's right in front of me.

I told my housekeeper that I was mouthing off on anything and everything in this book, and that I don't care who disagrees with me. Ruth is a woman who always speaks her mind. She said, "That's the advantage of getting old and dotty. You can say whatever you want and they have to listen." Old and dotty. Thanks, Ruth.

I don't expect to be "cured," in the normal sense. My melanoma is in me, and has been for at least twenty years. I asked my doctor about the word "remission." He told me that he doesn't use that word for Stage IV melanoma patients. The warped cells are rattling around inside me. The doctor can't predict when or where they'll gather enough strength to start their unchecked growth again. With medical help and the help of my own immune system, I may live long enough to die of something else before the melanoma whacks me. With any luck, it could be years. But the recent sighting of that small tumor in my butt is a warning that it could be a hell of a lot sooner.

The doctor said that dying of cancer does not usually result from the direct effects of a tumor acting on the body parts around it. He said that death comes because the body spends so much energy fighting the cancer that systems wear out and shut down. The person loses weight and gets weak and listless.

Although I've certainly had my moments, I am generally neither weak nor listless. That doesn't suit the personality of the Melanoma Mama. At the end of life, I know that some people welcome death as a way out of the struggle. I am nowhere near that point. I still spit in death's eye. I'm too busy sucking the juice out of life to be seduced by the Grim Reaper. Later, pal. Right now, take your scythe and your musty robe and your empty eye sockets and get lost!

I don't spend much time noodling over the subject of life after death. Frankly, I don't like the concept. It creeps me out. I'm hoping for complete lights out. I'm puzzled over the prevalence of the elaborate afterlives created by religions through the ages, and I'm disturbed by all the trouble their competing visions have caused. As my comedian friend, John Wetteland says, "A religious war is when people kill each other because they can't agree on what happens after we die."

Although I might remain in some people's memories after I die, I don't expect to lurk around in misty form to spook them. This said, I fully understand why so many people believe in ghosts. I experienced my father's presence after his death, and it was as vivid as if he had just walked through the door.

I was getting ready for work one morning, brushing my teeth. My father dropped in, in a friendly mood, as if to join me for breakfast. He was behind me to my right. His presence was so strong, that I turned to greet him. I felt a moment of eternity that lasted only a fraction of a second, then he was gone. I was happy to see him. It did not feel like a hallucination, and I knew I was not crazy. It seemed like the natural order of things. I remembered that he had died about one year earlier, so I asked my mother the exact date. It turns out that, without my remembering the date, I felt his presence precisely one year after he died.

When my grandmother was in her eighties, she told me that many years before, she had seen the ghost of a son who had died, and that she had never told anybody, because she was afraid they would deem her crazy and take her from her other children. But she knew she was not crazy. My brother also felt my deceased father pass through him. It was comforting to him.

These experiences feel real and are unexplainable scientifically, because you cannot predictably replicate them for scientific study. But even though I know the experience to be normal and to feel real, I cannot conclude that it proves my father's spirit returned from the dead. It was what it was. A mystery of love and of connection. It felt like an unexplainable rip in the fabric of space and time. Like entangled photons that, once together, are always together even when they've gone their separate ways.

I believe in the wonders of life right here and now. What fuels my hopeful spirit when I've got a ticking time bomb inside me? I rely on good doctors, wonderful friends and a supportive family. I rely on my body's proven resilience. When I was a child, there was a cartoon character called a Schmoo. It looked like a puffy bowling pin with a seal's face. I had a Schmoo toy–a large, plastic balloon, my own height. It was weighted at the bottom, so that, no matter how many times I punched the Schmoo to the floor, it came bouncing back up. Now I feel like that Schmoo. Punch me down, and I pop back up. At least I have so far. I'd prefer not to be punched so often, and I hate not knowing when the punch will be thrown, but so far I've bounced back.

One woman in my cancer support group was talking about the state of constant uncertainty that we late-stage patients must endure. She started off by saying, "I look up and I see ..." The way she rolled her eyes toward heaven, I thought she was going say she sees angels or the face of Jesus, but she said, "I see a little colored sneaker. You know, the other shoe that could drop at any time." I, too, walk beneath a colored sneaker that could drop at any time. Mine is pink and turquoise.

I promised an update on my recent diagnosis. The tumor in my butt was removed just before Christmas of 2009, and the plan was to use it make a vaccine. It didn't happen. I was all geared up for a four-month course of vaccine treatments, but they couldn't make the vaccine. Here is an email I sent friends and family about this part of my ongoing saga.

February 2, 2010: With any luck, this will be the last health update for a long time. I am now back to no treatments. We are simply watching and waiting with periodic scans. This is fine with me.

You may wonder what happened to the vaccine they were supposed to make from the tumor they carved from my butt. The bad news is they couldn't make the vaccine. But the good news is they couldn't make the vaccine. It's good news for two reasons.

First, they couldn't make it because there was hardly any melanoma in what they removed. Most of the tumor was my body's response to the little bit of melanoma that was there—I was walling it off and attacking it valiantly.

Second, when they tried to make the melanoma cells grow in order to make the vaccine, the cells up and died. This is good because, with aggressive forms of cancer, the cells proliferate without much coaxing. But my mel-

anoma cells are choosy—without just the right environment, they give up the ghost. I'm glad they're wimpy.

The doctor can't predict if or when another tumor
might crop up, but he assures me they have cutting-edge
treatments galore.

I've been enjoying some gorgeous days careening
down the slopes of Mt. Hood. Italian classes are getting
fun, although I'm still confusing Italian with Spanish.
They are deceptively similar. I'm just putting the finishing touches on the book I've been writing all fall. It's
called *Melanoma Mama.*

So now, I'm back to scans every three months. Watch and
wait. Watch and wait. Wait for the pink and turquoise sneaker to
drop. But I keep enjoying my miraculous recovery.

When I say miraculous, I don't mean a conventional
miracle. The radiation and the IL-2 explain much. Plus my
own body has proven trustworthy at keeping my melanoma at
bay for years. And if staying as healthy and happy as possible
boosts the immune system, then I'm doing my part. But just
because science can explain something, does not mean it's not
miraculous. It's miraculous that a Monarch butterfly can wing
its way from Canada to one small patch of breeding ground on
a Michoacan hillside. It's miraculous that a black hole's sucking
gravity can pull everything, including light into its gaping maw.
It's miraculous that there are billions of stars in our galaxy and
billions of galaxies in our universe. That my body can repair
itself while my brain isn't aware of the process—that's miraculous.

It's miraculous that I was born on a planet that wouldn't
have fostered life as we know it but for the fact that, early in
earth's history, an asteroid crashed into earth and chipped off
the moon, which ended up at just the right distance to hold
our orbit stable on its north-south axis, giving us predictable

seasons, which is needed for growing the plants we rely on; and that earlier still, our planet formed at just the right distance from the sun so that we neither freeze nor fry; and that earlier still, a nuclear reaction began cooking in the center of our sun. All the way back through time. One random chance after another. Cosmic collisions. One big chemistry lab in the sky. A wild physics experiment on a humongous scale. And somehow we're here.

And I'm still here, gazing with wonder at it all. This miracle. Humanity's fragile existence in the face of impossible odds is a deep wonder and the richest of treasures. So, yes. It's a miracle that the Melanoma Mama is still sucking air and dancing and singing.

So let's get the band together. Calling all you Melanoma Mamas out there. (If men join, we'll be the Melanoma Mamas and the Papas.) We'll make music, or at least we'll make a rowdy racket, and nobody will call us weak and listless. Not us. We'll start with, "Doctor, doctor, give me the news..." followed by, "Heaven can wait." So grab an instrument, and if you don't play, hum into a kazoo, and if you can't hum, tap out the beat with whatever is at hand—grab the doctor's stethoscope and tap it against your pain pole. Sing on key or off, but make sure you disturb the whole ward. Shake your bare booty in your backless johnny. We're not dead yet, and as long as we're here, let's be boisterously alive. When life and death no longer matter, true joy is possible.

◇◇◇◇◇

Where They Are Now

Cousin Ellen enjoys her retirement in Canada with Jake, Lulu, Cookie, and Muffin. Her breast cancer remains in remission.

Cousin Steve suffered a recurrence of his colon cancer and will remain on chemotherapy indefinitely, but he was able to go to the Philippines where he and his young bride Laarni renewed their vows at a lavish wedding ceremony.

Uncle Bill's diabetes wore him out. He failed to wake up on December 28, 2010 after celebrating Christmas with Steve, Laarni, Johnnice, and little Midgie.

Stepfather Frank died at home of a chronic lung disease on May 23, 2011. Until the end, he could look out his panoramic windows at his prize-winning flower garden.

Sister Catherine and her husband, Griff, love seeing deer and hearing owls at their home in rural Oregon. Sister Carol eats avocadoes from her backyard tree in Florida. Brother Chuck and his wife, Adrian are responsible worker bees in Massachusetts. Niece Elizabeth glories in theater and music.

Peder commutes from Oregon to Vietnam, but squeezes in wilderness adventures and romps with his family.

Nora spends October through February in Antarctica as a helicopter crew member at the main US science base, then returns to Wallowa, Oregon to ranch and to guide pack trips. Nora's peripatetic mother, Carol, was last spotted on a Moroccan camel.

Colleen valiantly teaches her exercise class three mornings a week in spite of a recurrence of her breast cancer.

Ann, the other Melanoma Mama, is still being monitored by Dr. Ernstoff and is still ebullient.

Both melanoma oncologists, Dr. Brendan Curti and Dr. Marc Ernstoff, remain chipper and optimistic. Dr. Curti's ongoing melanoma research on the combination of interleukin-2 with radiation is showing a dramatic success rate.

Many fine women in the cancer support group, *Making Today Count,* have come and gone. We pass the candle for each one who dies.

Mom, born in 1919, died tranquilly at home on October 21, 2011, one year after a lung cancer diagnosis. She enjoyed an eventful year in spite of being tethered to supplemental oxygen. She saw a book published which highlights her accomplishments as founder of a hiking group (*Over the Hill Hikers,* by Shirley Elder Lyons), and she won L.L. Bean's 2011 Outdoor Hero Award for her conservation work. She stood by Frank during his illness and death, and she embraced each day with humor and grace.

The Melanoma Mama: During all this time, the Incredible Shrinking Tumor kept shrinking, but my latest PET scan brought not such good news. Although it is not growing, the tumor shows up as a hot spot, meaning it was sucking nuclear-laced glucose like a vampire. So Dr. Curti is ready to start me on a year-long clinical trial where I will be injected with an immune-system booster called CT-011.

Two years ago, I enjoyed a dream-come-true trip to Italy where

I studied Italian in Lucca and in Florence. During this past year I was honored to be my mother's primary caregiver in New Hampshire. I also helped nurse my stepdad, Frank.

My books in progress are *Avoiding the Tuscan Sun - Melanoma Mama in Italy*, and *Life in the Slow Lane - Melanoma Mama as Caregiver*. The urgency of finishing my books has recently made itself clear. Medical drama abounds yet again.

On February 5, 2012, my sister Cathy and I were getting ready to go to the opera (Madame Butterfly) when she noticed that I was confused and uncoordinated. We didn't want to waste good opera tickets, so we went and enjoyed the performance. Then she took me to an emergency room where they performed a brain scan. The neurosurgeon, Dr. Deshmukh, said to me, "I have bad news." I felt my innards disappear. My only sensation was hollowness — a vast, uncertainty waiting to be filled with information. Inside that hollowness crouched the grim reaper, yet again. I knew life had just taken another of its unpredictable twists. Dr. D told me he saw a golf-ball-sized tumor in my right, frontal area and that he would remove it surgically. He admitted me to the hospital on the spot.

On Wednesday, February 8, 2012, Dr. D sawed into my forehead and sucked the tumor out with an aspirator. It was major surgery - more than four hours. There's a big hole inside which they tell me will fill up when brain cells grow back in there. Now, my scalp is stapled all along the hairline. The silver staples gleam, but, for glamour, I would prefer a rhinestone tiara.

It comes as no surprise that the biopsy of the tumor shows that it is melanoma. The doc assures me he got out what he needed to get out.

I awoke from the surgery alert and wanting to get out of bed and walk around. I have been walking short distances each day. They sent me home to my sister's care only two days after the surgery. Now I'm in my home with plenty of help from friends.

For support, I have life-long friends in Oregon plus dozens of get-well cards from friends in NH. I have my cancer support group, Making Today Count. I have my writing. I watch movies and I eat ice cream. Life is still rich and full, but Dr. D forbids me to ski for at least six months. Spoilsport.

Did I see this brain surgery coming? Two weeks prior I had been to a four-day dance retreat (improvisation) at which we danced many hours a day. I felt somewhat sluggish, but enjoyed the retreat. I had been having symptoms of forgetfulness, disorganization and such, but we all attributed my low mental functioning to my grief over Mom's death. So except for some headaches and some intermittent earaches, I was blindsided by this huge honkin' brain tumor.

So here's the bad news and the good news. Bad news: you can be having a normal, enjoyable day, and they can announce that you must take a detour for brain surgery. Good news: They can suck a golf-ball out of your brain and leave you with most of what you need to function.

I log my progress on my journal at Caring Bridge (http://www.caringbridge.org/visit/melanomamama). That's how to keep track of me.

◇◇◇◇◇

About the Author

Constance Emerson Crooker, a Stage IV melanoma patient, spends time in both Oregon and New Hampshire. She attends *Making Today Count*, a women's cancer support group at Providence Hospital in Oregon.

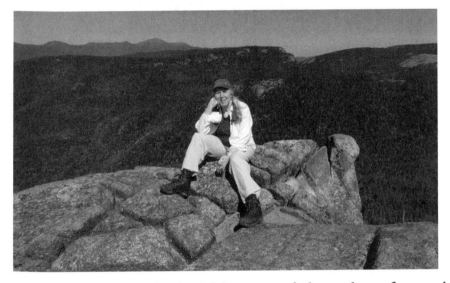

Constance is a retired trial lawyer and the author of several law-related books including *Gun Control and Gun Rights*. She has written numerous articles for an eclectic range of periodicals from legal (*Champion, Oregon State Bar Bulletin, Oregon Defense Attorney*) to outdoor (*AMC Outdoors, Appalachia*) to popular (*High Times*) to academic (*Reed Magazine*). Her opinions have appeared in articles in *The New York Times* and *The Oregonian*.

Constance teaches creative writing techniques in Connie's Writing Playground and she speaks at writing conferences on the business of writing.

She is working on two more Melanoma Mama books. Watch

for the upcoming *Avoiding the Tuscan Sun–Melanoma Mama in Italy* and *Life in the Slow Lane–Melanoma Mama as Caregiver.*

www.melanomamama.com

How to Help

Ten percent of the profits from the sale of Melanoma Mama's books will go to melanoma research. If you wish to join in contributing, send donations to:

Make checks payable to:
Norris Cotton Cancer Center–Melanoma Research

Mail to:
Norris Cotton Cancer Center–Melanoma Research
Dartmouth-Hitchcock/DMS Development Office
1 Medical Center Drive
Lebanon, NH 03756

For further information: (603)653-0743

And/or:

Make checks payable to:
Melanoma Cancer Research

Mail to:
Providence Portland Medical Foundation
4805 NE Glisan Street
Portland, Oregon 97213

For further information: (503) 215-6187